For the millions of people struggling to escape their own compulsions, **Obsessive-Compulsive Disorders** is a landmark on the path to recovery

△

"Addresses with great wisdom, tremendous experience, and enviable success the treatment of obsessive-compulsive behaviors.... This book is filled with common sense."
—Samuel Klagsburn, M.D., Medical Director
Four Winds Hospital, Katonah, New York

△

"Outstanding!...He has indeed made a great contribution in discovering and sharing with such clarity the effective treatment approach for these diseases."
—Raymond E. Vath, M.D., P.S.,
Clinical Assistant Professor
Department of Psychiatry, University of Washington

△

"For recovering alcoholics and addicts, as well as counselors and therapists, this book sheds light on the underlying issues that must be confronted to achieve recovery as a total person."
—Carol Cox Smith, M.A.Ed., author of
Recovery at Work: A Clean and Sober Career Guide

△

Also by Steven Levenkron

Kessa

Treating and Overcoming Anorexia Nervosa

The Best Little Girl in the World

OBSESSIVE-COMPULSIVE DISORDERS

D I S O R D E R S

TREATING AND UNDERSTANDING CRIPPLING HABITS

STEVEN LEVENKRON

WARNER BOOKS

A Time Warner Company

To the memory of my mother,
Florence Levenkron

While the stories presented in this book are drawn from actual cases, all of the names and any identifying characteristics concerning the individuals depicted in the stories have been changed to make them wholly unrecognizable to protect their identity and privacy.

Copyright © 1991 by Steven Levenkron
All rights reserved.
Warner Books, Inc., 666 Fifth Avenue, New York, NY 10103

W A Time Warner Company
Printed in the United States of America
First Trade Printing: January 1992
10 9 8 7 6 5 4 3 2 1

Library of Congress Cataloging-in-Publication Data
Levenkron, Steven, 1941-
   Obsessive-compulsive disorders : treating and understanding crippling habits / Steven Levenkron.
      p.   cm.
   Includes bibliographical references and index.
   ISBN 0-446-39348-7
   I. Obsessive-compulsive disorder—Popular works.   I. Title.
RC533.L48   1991
616.85′227—dc20   90-50280
                                                              CIP

Book design by Giorgetta Bell McRee
Cover design by Judith Kadzyn Leeds

ACKNOWLEDGMENTS

I would like to thank my wife, Abby, who as my co-therapist and editor of the first manuscript draft, helped with this undertaking. My thanks also go to Buck Biggers for his editorial skills in the final organization of the manuscript. A special thanks to Susan Suffes at Warner, who has been the kind of editor writers only hope to work with. She has been as much a supportive collaborator as an editor.

CONTENTS

Introduction

In the years following the publication of my book *Treating and Overcoming Anorexia Nervosa,* I have received calls from individuals who stated that they suffered from all the feelings that characterize persons with eating disorders: they were compulsive about daily routines and good at nurturing others but were unable to feel close to them; they found it difficult to accept care and suffered continuously from feelings of emptiness. They asked if they could be treated for these problems and wanted to know if there was a name for what was wrong with them. Often the caller asked if he or she belonged to a diagnostic category. I indicated that while I didn't think they ought to be labeled and placed in a formal diagnostic category, I would informally term the group of problems they complained about "obsessional disorders."

While many callers actually suffered from obsessive-compulsive disorders, others simply had to think repeatedly about everything they did. It is this excessive "overthinking" that I call obsessional. An obsessional disorder might be characterized not by symptoms or moods but by particular behaviors employed to control anxiety and depression. These behaviors are self-soothing and they are used by individuals who are unable to accept comfort and support from others.

The callers were identifying with those suffering from eating disorders; some were even "recovering" eating-disorder victims themselves. That particular group complained that their eating disorders had been treated, almost "exorcised," but they still didn't feel good. Some even claimed to feel worse since they didn't have a way to focus bad feelings the way they used to—on eating and weight. While some protested about the behavior-modification programs that stopped their eating disorders, others were critical about the years of fruitless analytical psychotherapy that had left them feeling as empty as it had found them. And those who never had eating disorders made all the same complaints about themselves, their moods and their limitations, as those who did. It became obvious to me, from my particular vantage point, that all of these people had much in common with each other and that one way to identify this commonality was to see all of these problems as part of "obsessional disorders." The second and more important task, was to conceptualize a way to treat people in this kind of pain.

While much has been written about obsessive-compulsive disorders, or OCD, as a neurological defect—where something is wrong with the brain—I see OCD as the personality's attempt to reduce anxiety, which may stem from a painful childhood or a genetic tendency toward anxiety that just won't quit. As I thought more about the victims of OCD I have treated, it seems that a major factor in their progress has been their ability to use me as a mediator of their impulses and as someone to whom the unthinkable could be said. It is this aspect of treatment that I would like to focus on in treating and understanding the crippling habits that are known as obsessive-compulsive disorders.

The individual who takes care of himself when there is no one else available is adapting to his situation. However, if he is never able to depend upon others, or receive comfort and support from them when they *are* available, then he is mistrust-ful, despairing of the value of others to be of help. The aim of this book is to assist those charged with treating the mistrustful and to assist those suffering from obsessional disorders.

—S. L.

ONE

Obsessive-Compulsive Disorders

My daughter desperately needs help," said the woman who sat before me, the fifteen-year-old subject of her conversation sitting resolutely in the chair beside her. "Olivia showers for at least an hour and a half every night. After that, she will arrange her books for an hour before she can begin her homework. When her homework is complete—at about midnight—she starts the selection of her next day's clothing, a process that has her going over and over almost everything she owns, so that the selection continues to God knows what hour." The mother shook her head. "It breaks my heart to wake her up in the morning knowing she's had only a few hours' sleep. I just can't understand what's the matter with her."

Olivia suffers from obsessive-compulsive disorder (OCD), a pervasive condition that causes individuals to overexamine their thoughts, spoken words, actions, productivity, and relationships. In this overexamination, they always find what they have done—whether words, thoughts, or actions—inadequate and wanting. This mental examination process is repeated over and over throughout the day, often generating a dangerous level of tension. They are never satisfied with themselves. Rarely, if ever, are they happy.

They repeat their activities with an intensity bordering on desperation. Many of us have seen them . . .

▲ Running fifteen miles a day in rain or shine, without training for anything specific.

▲ Working twelve hours a day, six or seven days a week, yet feeling they are getting nowhere.

▲ Shopping endlessly and buying many more items than they can possibly use.

▲ Showering for two hours a day, changing clothes repeatedly, yet never feeling clean.

▲ Searching day in and day out for items they never get around to using or for clothes they forget to wear.

We see examples of this behavior in those we live with rather than those we work with, for it is behavior people are more apt to do at home and away from work and public position. This behavior is confusing; we see the intensity and repetition and it puzzles us.

Sometimes we inquire, "Why do you do that so often? Why do you do that so intensely?"

The answer is usually, "Oh, you don't understand. I just don't feel good unless I do this the way I do."

What they cannot tell us (for they do not know) is that these repeated activities, or rituals, are actually self-soothing devices used to fill an emotional emptiness caused by underparenting or impaired receptivity to parenting in early childhood. These repeated activities are pacifiers now called upon because the parent figure needed much earlier—a loving, trusted, authoritative parent—was either missing or weakened or depleted, often so much so that the result was role reversal for parent and child.

Unable to depend upon a strong parent figure, individuals like Olivia turn inward, learning to depend upon their own invented behaviors. So twisted does this dependency become, that as the obsessive-compulsive rituals continue and proliferate, these young people move into total isolation, unable to reach out to *anyone.*

Underparenting is on the rise in this nation, and so is OCD. During the past ten years, the number of reported cases has increased alarmingly, and this rate of increase is almost certain to accelerate in the decade ahead. We live in an age when millions of parents are so obsessed with making money that they do not have enough time or energy for proper child care, an age when the drive for a fashionable image defined by expensive cars and opulent homes, designer clothes, and flawless faces and figures has driven couples into modes of thinking and ways of living that are separating parents from their children much too early. This style of living prevents them from ever being close enough; often mothers feel that caring for their children is the lowest part of their day in terms of self-esteem. And this lifestyle teaches career women that it's very nice to have children, but to make certain they don't get caught on the Mommy track.

All this is disastrous for the nurturing quality in our nation. Perceiving society as nonsupportive to motherhood, many women become conflicted in their mothering behavior. They resent the draining demands that work, marriage, and motherhood produce. And if they become convinced that motherhood is something to be ashamed of, then their children will not have the experience of support, commitment, and caretaking as part of childhood.

Fathers, on the other hand, traditionally feel more justified in devoting themselves to the world of work. But at home they often feel distant, left out, and unappreciated, lacking any real authority. Children have always required focus and authority as well as love from their parents. Today's emotionally beleaguered parents often have more difficulty with authoritative behavior and focus than with love.

In families where the mother holds a full-time job, she often returns to work within just two months of delivery, considerably less time than most West European nations allot for the postnatal leave of absence. With societal pressure on women to compete vigorously with men in careers and still be identified as the primary parent, underparenting is the inevitable result. This means more and more young people struggling with emotional isolation, unable to depend upon anyone or anything but their extraordinary rituals—rituals like the ones that had brought teenage Olivia and her mother to my office.

"Sometimes I don't know Olivia at all," her mother told me now. "I hope you can help her."

I turned to the daughter, an attractive, well-dressed young lady. Only the darkness beneath her eyes offered evidence that something was wrong. Looking a bit belligerantly at her mother, she said, "I don't need anyone's help. I have everything under control." Then she turned to me. "I think my mother means well, but I'm a methodical person, that's all. Maybe I'm a perfectionist, but that's better than being a slob."

Ignoring the implied insult, her mother said, "Don't you admit you spend too much time in the shower?"

"No, Mother, I don't. I shower until I'm clean. That's all. I'm a neat, organized person. There's nothing bad about that."

Olivia's neatness and organization extended far beyond the normal. Almost every moment of her waking life was devoted to some sort of ritual. The showers, the book arranging, the clothing choice, touching parts of her body before dressing, and finger counting required so much time and energy that she was being forced deeper and deeper into herself, into withdrawal and isolation. So complex and pervasive were these rituals that Olivia was often unable to attend school because she had fallen behind in her rituals and had to stay home so she could complete her mental list from the previous day!

When alone with her mother or father, if confronted with the overwhelming power of her repetitious behavior and asked even for a modest show of improvement, she would burst into temper tantrums, shouting denunciations and accusations.

"She seems like a monster then," her mother told me privately. "Somebody I don't know anymore. If only she'd stop some of the repetition."

* * *

What is the magic of repetition? Why is it so appealing as a self-soothing device for the obsessional personality? Repetition brings familiarity, and familiarity is the opposite of the unknown. Repetition is there in our earliest, most natural self-soothing action: sucking. When an infant becomes distressed, it sucks at the breast or bottle.

And sucking, this first and most basic form of repetition, is much more than simply soothing. It is our instinctive way to obtain nutrition. It is also our first social act, for it begins as an activity with Mother. Once the period of nursing is past, the benefits of repetition alone become even more obvious as self-soothing is sought in thumb or pacifier. There is no milk here, no social contact, only repetition and familiarity.

Consider the repetition in other childhood forms of self-soothing activity: clutching a cherished baby blanket, hugging a worn teddy bear, listening to the same story read night after night (and don't dare change the ending), watching TV cartoons again and again. Repetition is familiar, familiar is predictable, and predictable is safe.

The form or forms this repetition takes in the obsessional child will depend upon the particular remedy the child seizes upon to reduce his or her level of anxiety. For example, if some authority figure has warned the child to be certain hands are washed before dinner or after using the bathroom, the child may invent an inner voice saying, "Wash your hands." And this can be the beginning of an obsessive-compulsive structure. If the structure works—providing at least momentary calmness or some lessening of anxiety—this ritual will be reinforced; that is, the individual's mind will say, "Handwashing helped handle the anxiety, so it must be a good thing to do." Repeated handwashing immediately becomes a proven ritual, and the broad base of cleanliness may be expanded and complicated.

Linda, a twenty-two-year-old patient, explained her bathroom rituals this way: "I have to wash my hands before touching my clothes; and before washing my hands, I have to tear off a one-foot length of toilet paper and remove two paper towels from the dispenser. If it's a cloth towel dispenser, I pull out nearly two feet of it. Sometimes I wash my hands before and after this part. If I check the door lock, I have to wash my hands again. I always line the toilet seat with either a regular liner or toilet paper in case I inadvertently sit on the seat. I try to avoid that, though. I use a lot of toilet paper when I'm finished, then I wait a minute or two and use more. Now I have to wash my hands again before touching myself or my clothes. After I'm finished with my clothes, I wash my hands again. I have to turn off the water faucets by holding them with paper towels. I need a new paper towel to open the door. If I touch the faucets or the doorknob with my hand, I have to wash again until I get it right. Sometimes I get so frustrated I could scream, but I can't disobey the rules."

Linda mentioned that she did not like to enter a bathroom unless she could allow herself at least a half hour within, so she often waited hours after she realized she needed to use the bathroom until a suitable opportunity could be found.

When the time comes that the handwashing and other bathroom rituals fail to provide sufficient relief from anxiety, the individual looks for another behavior pattern to follow. Perhaps the memory calls up, "Be sure the door is locked." And checking the door locks becomes a second safe-making device. Should these two rituals eventually fail to provide sufficient relief from anxiety, even when expanded and repeated many times, a third activity may be added. Then a fourth and fifth and so on. Since the aim is simply to make one feel less anxious, this self-soothing process knows no bounds except time.

Of course, we all need self-soothing devices at some point in our lives, especially as children. If our parents leave our bedroom, perhaps turning out the light, fears close in like wolves on a lost lamb. We reach into the darkness for something to comfort us, some familiar "friend"—a thumb, a pacifier, a blanket, a teddy bear. We find it, and the darkness becomes bearable.

All this is normal. But one day these self-soothing devices

must be surrendered. We must learn to face the darkness, the unknown, without a crutch. And it is not always easy. Remember Gene Wilder's character desperately hanging on to his blue blanket in the movie *The Producers?* Or Linus clinging to his in the comic strip *Peanuts?* These reassuring objects must be surrendered if we are to mature normally and develop inner character.

What enables a child to make the break? How does he or she find the strength to risk the unfamiliar and unpredictable? Through the continuing encouragement of a strong parent (sometimes a grandparent or nanny) on whom the child can depend and in whom he or she has complete trust. This person's reassurance and encouragement will make the unfamiliar feel safe or, at least, tolerable. Their strength and authority will give the child someone to lean on and depend upon. And normal emotional growth can take place.

When such a parent is not available or is too weak or ill to play a sufficient role in the child's life or is abruptly taken from the child by departure or death, the result is underparenting, and the voyage toward normal emotional maturity may be aborted. And if at some point in the future the child's level of anxiety rises to a point that is unbearable, what is he or she to do? Denied adequate support, there is no inner strength or emotional maturity upon which to draw. There is only a sense of emptiness that the child will struggle to fill with some sort of reassuring conduct, conduct that by its mere repetition is calming, much as the words of a person loved and depended upon might be calming.

Although children cling to supportive statements, they also cling to critical ones, words that indicate they are the keen focus of their parents. Thus the underparented child, searching for some reassuring conduct, might imagine his parents instructing him to clean his bedroom. The child then invents a voice saying, "Clean up your room." And the ritual has begun. (The paradox here is that at some point the parents will take great pride in their child's being a "self-starter" and keeping things clean independently, never recognizing that the child is obsessionally and repeatedly directing himself to keep his room clean in order to replace the strong parental instructions he secretly longs for.)

The severity of the underparenting will determine the severity of the child's rituals, ranging from barely noticeable to outrageous: endless handwashing and showering; constant cleaning or rearranging of objects; repeated checking of door locks, buttons, zippers, stove knobs, or virtually any object. And repetitious, obsessional thinking is characteristic of the problem.

Twenty-three-year-old Ashley used exercise for her long list of rituals. She often stood in my waiting room prior to her appointment and "paced a mile." She also ran three miles a day. In addition, she followed a rigorous videotaped workout and swam for a half hour at her health club. She never took a bus if she had time to walk. She walked at twice the pace of most of us. During a therapy session, she would flex muscles in her arms and legs continuously. Her knuckles would whiten from the intensity of the fist she was making while resting her hands on the arms of the chair.

"I can stop worrying about most things when I know all my exercises are in place," she told me. "If they're not, I feel required to worry. I worry about school, my brothers, my parents. If I don't actively think about them, I feel something terrible will happen to them. I know that sounds crazy, but if I haven't done my exercises, I feel safer when I'm worried; worrying is one of my rituals."

Ashley explained that she felt most secure when all her obligations were completed for the day. In fact, she identified herself as "someone who fulfills obligations."

"If I do what is obligatory, I am safe."

I inquired, "Who decides just what is obligatory?"

"I do."

"How do you decide?"

"I don't know how each requirement started. It usually started as an extension of some other requirement. For example, my running started at two miles a day, once I got in shape.

Then I added a half mile if I thought I did something wrong for that day. Soon my basic requirement was up to three miles a day as well as other exercises if I felt something was wrong. I figure that all in all, I do two hours of intense exercise every day."

"Do you have other obligations?"

She laughed nervously. "Zillions of them."

"Could you tell me what some of them are?"

"Well, one or two of them stem from running, at least they came after I started running—I think. When I run, I sweat . . ." She laughed nervously again. ". . . so I have to shower. Well, I shower like I do everything else. It takes me a half hour to shower, and to protect that investment of time and to avoid a second or third shower, or fourth in the summer, I change my underwear frequently, every three hours, if I can." There was a pause. "Do you think that underwear changing has some special significance?"

"How do you feel when you've just put on clean underwear?"

"The same way I feel when I've run three miles. I feel like I've completed an important obligation . . . for now, relieved."

"Does completion of an obligation always make you feel relieved?"

"Sometimes the relief is only partial."

"What does that mean?"

"It depends on how often I have to repeat it."

"Then there *is* partial relief?"

"It's hard to explain to anyone. If I'm doing one exercise, and I know it's part of a set that I'll have to repeat, I just feel, well, so far so good. When I check the locks on my apartment door the first time, I know it's just the beginning, and I know I won't feel right until I've checked them at least three times. While I'm touching them, I'm feeling relaxed, but the minute I stop, I feel anxious again. I actually lose sight of the reason for checking them. I get so into the act and the repetition it's almost like being in a trance. I just get into the rhythm of it. It doesn't matter anymore whether I think the door is secure. I just want to continue handling the knob, pushing the door, turning the key in the locking direction. Sometimes it feels like the repetition could go on forever, and then I remind myself that I'm on my way out of the house, and I make myself stop."

Once the individual becomes accustomed to this method of relieving anxiety and the rituals begin to proliferate, an inventory process becomes an essential part of the pattern. Keeping track of the expanding system of rituals eventually requires continuous thinking and rethinking. Only through such constant checking can the individual be certain all the rituals have been performed: hands washed both twice before and after using the bathroom; front and back door locks checked three times each; books placed in alphabetical, size, or use order, then checked several times to be certain the order is correct; clothes prepared for the next day, sweaters counted, checked for stains, placed in a drawer, then taken out and recounted, rechecked, then replaced in the drawer, then taken out and recounted, rechecked, then placed in the drawer again; it doesn't stop.

This repetitive behavior is almost always accompanied by obsessional thinking—the overexamination of details beyond the point of reasonable attention. Imagine the time that goes into such thinking and such rituals! No wonder the obsessive-compulsive person has little time or energy left for others. He or she withdraws socially, not so much because of antisocial tendencies, but because the internal mental business is so demanding.

"I'm going to get an answering machine," nineteen-year-old Katharine told me. "That way I won't have to talk with my friends anymore."

"Why?" I asked. "What priorities do you have that you don't have time for your friends?"

"My priorities are not people. People just get in the way."

"Get in the way of what?" I asked.

"All the rituals I have to do. There are particular ways of getting out of bed, special ways of using the bathroom, washing, making meals, cleaning the apartment, exercising, getting ready to go shopping. I'm so busy that it's difficult to get them all done each day."

"Do you wonder why you have to do all these rituals?"

"No. They're all just imperative. It's unthinkable not to do them."

"What would you feel like if you didn't?"

She thought a moment, looking nervous even as the prospect was considered. "I would feel very, very tense," she told me finally. "And I would continue feeling very, very tense until what I was supposed to do was done. I couldn't stand that."

Since nothing else seems to reduce the person's level of anxiety, he or she becomes totally dependent on the rituals, so emotionally isolated that reaching out for help or accepting it when offered is almost impossible.

This, then, is the structure of obsessive-compulsive disorders:

ANATOMY OF OCD

1. Continuous anxiety state due to either biological-hereditary or environmental causes.
2. Concern that parents are unable to make one feel better.
3. Development of a sense of hopelessness about depending on others for comfort, support, and guidance.
4. Emotionally turning inward; feeling disconnected from others.
5. Inventing secret pseudosolutions (rituals) for resolution of emotional distress.
6. Discarding emotional accessibility due to intense belief in rituals and preoccupation (obsession) with carrying them out.

Since these rituals must be repeated to head off more anxiety, they are *compulsive*. And since the person must overthink each ritual in order to make certain it is performed both properly and adequately, thinking becomes *obsessive*. It is for these reasons that this disorder, this particular combination of thought and behavior is termed *obsessive-compulsive disorder*.

It is nothing to trifle with. Left untreated, it will, at best, offer a weary life filled with meaningless rituals and void of meaningful relationships. At worst, it often spirals downward into physical conduct that becomes life-threatening.

Twenty-five years ago, cultural changes pointed toward a reduction in obsessive-compulsive disorders. Today, precisely the opposite is true. We have entered the Obsessional Age, and unless major cultural changes are forthcoming quickly, we could witness explosive growth in the number of people suffering from OCD.

TWO

The Age of Obsession

Is there a way to stem this tide? A decrease in obsessive-compulsive disorders depends upon an increase in proper parental nurturing. Such a decrease requires men and women who are ready for long-term commitment as parents, putting the good of their children first, often subjugating their own needs and desires to those of their offspring. In the 1960s and, to a lesser extent, the 1970s, signs were encouraging. A caring society is more likely to produce caring parents, and everywhere there was an air of altruism.

Social issues connected people across class and racial lines. Members of the white middle class were involved in the civil rights movement. Many traveled south and joined in dangerous marches. White youths in the north picketed local Woolworth stores because "Southern Woolworths Segregate at the Lunch Counter," as the placards read. Thousands of whites joined Martin Luther King's march on Washington.

Social struggles became the subject of contemporary songs, such as Bob Dylan's incisive ballads "Only a Pawn in Their Game" and "The Lonesome Death of Hattie Carol," which dealt with race and poverty. "Masters of War" and "The Times They

Are A-Changin'" later came to reflect the moral outrage many Americans shared about the nation's involvement in Vietnam. The tone of the Woodstock Generation was one of caring, sharing, and social involvement.

As for the specific nurturing of children, lectures and magazine articles addressed underparenting by fathers and talked about a fuller two-parent family. Women joined consciousness-raising groups for peer support and self-understanding; some men formed similar groups. Women began to see maternity leave as another civil right for which to struggle. Breast-feeding came out of the closet and onto park benches, and there was a pride on the part of mothers in their ability to biologically nurture their children.

Women began to feel that physicians were coming between them and their infants in the birth process. Lamaze and other natural-childbirth techniques entered the delivery room along with fathers. Obstacles to nurturing were pushed aside. Gynecologists and pediatricians had their consciousness raised by newly alert mothers. Young fathers were seen in the streets carrying their babies in specially designed infant carriers strapped close to their bodies, and toddlers rode in backpacks. It was an exciting time to be a parent. Pregnancy, childbirth, and nursing one's child provided status.

Today, all of that has changed. Unlike the time of caring and nurturing that was enjoyed in the 1960s, the 1980s proved to be a time of self-reliance or, less charitably, self-centeredness. If a caring society is more likely to produce caring parents, then the opposite must also be true. And consider the track record of the 1980s.

Under conservative government stewardship, the public sector had diminished its financial support for schools and child care. And public attitudes supported this diminishing of the caretaking activities of government. Directly or indirectly, Americans voted for reductions in public spending on child care, education, and the needy. And it may be inferred that the more financially fortunate are losing interest in the problems of the less fortunate.

Meanwhile, the culture of consumerism and the market economy has devalued family relationships. Corporate take-overs, motivated by greed, have demoralized workers, for employees are demeaned if their job security exists only as it suits owner needs. When corporations are purchased for the property value of profitable production plants, and these plants or stores are then shut down in order to make a property sale, there is not only a financial ripple in terms of mass firings, but a psychological aftereffect as well. And when breadwinners are dispensable, regardless of their productivity, the demoralization process is felt through the family structure. The tension and distress affect parenting. If parents are demoralized by economic insecurity, their ability to nurture their children is limited, and often they are more in need of comforting themselves.

As the air of materialism blows throughout our land, relationships to others have become less valued than the ways we measure ourselves, especially in terms of our purchasing power. Men postpone marriage and fatherhood in favor of financial success or security, then feel handicapped and angry when children arrive. Competing with men in the job market, many women are ashamed of their biological femininity and fearful of pregnancy. When it occurs, they resent the child and, fearing for their job future, return to work just weeks after birth, delivering the child over to a nanny or some form of day care. The chance for divorce is increased by the strain of two-career marriages, and this produces yet more divided parenting, more nannies, more day care.

For that section of the urban population where married women have been trained to be as ambitious as their husbands, and no allowance is made for pregnancy, childbirth and child care, women are experiencing a double burden that puts them in continuous conflict from the time they become pregnant until the time they deliver and go back to work. While this will affect the urban portion of married women most intensely, the ripple effect, as a cultural trend, will affect most women who see themselves as career-oriented.

A recent *Newsweek* poll shows that an astonishing two-thirds of all mothers and more than half of all mothers of infants are in the work force. There is nothing in the culture that is supportive right now for child raising by mothers. And this lack of support creates a pressure that results in underparenting on the part of biological mothers with a career focus. It is this heightened anxiety on the part of mothers—and especially the new mothers—that creates anxious parenting, which may be received by the child as *resentful* parenting.

With all this lessening of the quality of child nurture, we seem destined for an explosion in the number of obsessive-compulsive disorders. But we act as if we cannot wait for this explosion to occur. Like lemmings buying beachwear, we herald the Age of Obsession by romanticizing the concept. How much marketing research went into the naming of the Calvin Klein perfume Obsession? How many new articles, books, and films have "Obsession" in their titles? How many others like *Fatal Attraction* have obsession at the core of the plot even though it is not in the title?

Our focus on obsession is part of our daily lives. The sense of well-being once found in the development of relationships is now found (or searched for) by many in an obsession with some form of self-improvement, such as dieting or exercise. One has only to watch the athletes training and performing in the international Olympic Games to see examples of obsessiveness as a motivator, driving people to achieve body perfection. And although this behavior and attitude is reasonable within the context of intense athletic competition, such intense drives are not normal or appropriate in everyday life. Yet consider the increasing number of adults obsessed with running and jogging, aerobics, and exercise machines. Many articles have been published identifying "obligatory runners' syndrome" and "compulsive exercising."

Obsessing about one's own physical perfection has led many to fixate on the physical perfection of a potential partner. The once separate exercising facilities for men and women have become combined so that the quest for the perfect mate becomes the search for the perfect body, which has nothing to do with real relationships. Out of this body search comes a kind of social and sexual compulsive promiscuity, involving continuous attracting, evaluating, and rejecting of prospective mates. As in any obsessive ritual, the goal is not to solve the problem, but to perpetuate the need for the repetitious behavior. In the case of compulsive promiscuity, fault finding is the goal. So the compulsive-promiscuous person can never designate anyone as adequate lest the obsessive process of searching (fault finding) comes to a halt.

The process of video screening of possible dates and mates simply adds to the mechanical nature of this procedure, and it is something one can do literally in isolation so it becomes one more way to perpetuate obsessive promiscuity.

As the health clubs and the singles bars and the video clubs become arenas for personal rejection and failed attempts at attachments, marketing strategists in advertising extol independence as the new virtue in the Age of Obsession. For example, a perfume company marketed its product by showing a woman driving her sports car to the seashore to watch the sunset by herself. One cannot help but wonder why the sponsor stressed using the perfume to be alone?

If it is not improving our body about which we are obsessing, it may be improving the number and quality of our possessions, as evidenced by endless shopping trips or, in the case of the new TV home shopping channels, day or night calls on the telephone. Indeed, the act of purchasing something has become well recognized as self-soothing behavior for the Age of Obsession. On a July 1989 episode of the TV soap opera *Loving*, a mother let her daughter know that she was worried about the young woman's depression, especially in view of the suicidal tendencies she had previously demonstrated. The young woman responded flippantly, "I'm going to do the only thing a totally depressed, suicidal person *can* do. I'm going to shop and shop until I feel good again."

Items that thirty years ago were regarded as luxuries are today considered by most Americans to be necessities. Much of what is being manufactured today might be termed the Obsession Market: goods that are purchased not because they are needed, but because acquiring them makes the buyer feel cared for. Advertisements promise "that pampered feeling." Cosmetics top the list, but they also include electronic toys and expensive-looking watches for men and women. These kinds of goods are found on the first floor of the major department stores to snare potential purchasers. One can see all this in the purchasing and spending so characteristic of the Yuppie Generation (and so constantly encouraged by the commercial sector and media advertising).

Thorstein Veblen's concept of conspicuous consumption is familiar to many of us. He identified the acquisition of expensive goods, especially jewelry and furs by rich men's wives, as a sign to others that their husbands were successful. In the Age of Obsession, conspicuous consumption has different emotional overtones. Luxury goods are advertised to a broader economic group, and those who will have to struggle to buy expensive automobiles or status-offering condos are encouraged to do so in order to look (and feel) financially and socially adequate. The pressure to look well off goes so far down the economic spectrum that those who cannot possibly afford a Mercedes are encouraged to buy an automobile with a similar profile and look-alike logo.

The message is no longer conspicuous consumption but adequacy consumption. We no longer buy to prove we are a success, we spend to prove we are not a failure. Like the Olympic athlete, members of the American middle class are competing to be seen as winners, but even more to avoid being seen as losers. With the same obsessionality that the athlete brings to focus upon musculature, coordination, timing, and stamina for a particular event, the middle-class person may have to ward off fears of "falling behind the Joneses."

A society where one is expected to afford the lifestyle advertised in the Sunday *New York Times Magazine* is a society where most members must inevitably feel financially inadequate; and the only way to become acceptable is to earn and spend more. As the middle class becomes increasingly obsessed by the fear of inadequacy, like the obsessionally disordered individual, a sense of desperate emptiness develops. And just as an individual's obsessive-compulsive behavior has caused him to neglect identity development (personal reflection, relationships, attachments, and intimacies), the obsessional status seeker creates the same personality deficit in the race to escape inadequacy by spending money. As one becomes accustomed to spending money to relieve feelings of inadequacy, the act of spending, over time, becomes a security-making ritual, not unlike handwashing for the compulsive cleaner.

More important, however, than these acts in themselves (or their place as signposts in the Age of Obsession) is what they eventually lead to in terms of inadequate parenting. Fear of not having enough money, for example, is often responsible for the postponement of marriage and parenthood, and the putting off of having children until it can be "done right," meaning until one is on sound financial ground and all the material goods are in place. But how much financial health is enough in today's society? Is security an impossible goal in the Age of Obsession? Many men approach marriage as something necessary, even wished for, but nonetheless threatening.

This feeling often begins early; perhaps it starts when college men tell their dates, "I have my future to think of. I can't get involved at this stage of my life." This now-popular campus litany, heard by many a coed as the reason for ending a budding relationship, certainly puts young women on notice. The message is clear: You're on your own. Don't expect proposals of marriage from this group.

Once men learn this litany, can they ever unlearn it? Women frequently report the same statements from men in their thirties. In "Whether to Marry," an August 1988 *New York Times Magazine* article, the author indicated that many men become locked into avoidance of intimacy and are more attracted to the obsessions (such as exercise) that are part of their well-developed isolation.

Aware of men's distaste for or fear of marriage, women learn to disguise their own desires for marriage and motherhood. Even their language about this is guarded.

("We're getting serious," a young woman recently commented to me in regard to a man she was seeing.

When I asked how serious, she answered, "We're considering making a long-term commitment." A moment later, as I remained silent, she added, "A permanent one."

I thought I understood, but to make certain, I asked, "Do you mean marriage?"

"Oh yes," she said. "Of course." But she looked around as if afraid of being overheard.)

Marriage is a word many women have learned to avoid. For those of us currently in middle age, this is an extreme swing of the societal pendulum. Twenty years ago, it was necessary for women to be free from the belief that to be a complete person they needed to be married. Now that the cultural emphasis has turned against marriage, and even encourages a woman to feel ashamed of her desire (no matter how healthy the desire may be), that aspect of the cultural message is unhealthy.

When a man and woman do marry, fear of financial inadequacy continues to play a major role in shaping their lives. First of all, there is the question of whether or not the woman should give up her job to become a full-time mother. Not only would this mean the loss of one income, it would also mean, in the eyes of many, a demotion for the wife. According to a guest on the Phil Donahue show in November 1988, child care is considered "a job with very low status." Indeed, taking care of children, especially in ambitious urban circles, has become synonymous with being left behind. This issue was addressed in the 1972 film *Up the Sandbox!* starring Barbra Streisand. The story depicts an intelligent married woman discovering that her social status was deteriorating because she was staying home to raise her children. She goes to parties attended by high-powered career women. One tells her, "I might do the kid thing for a year or so." During the course of the story, the Streisand character sees her self-esteem slipping away as a result of full-time motherhood.

Made from Anne Roiphe's insightful novel, the film illustrates one half of the painful conflict women experience when
choosing between motherhood and the marketplace. Coupled
with the other half—fear of financial inadequacy—this is often
enough to make women of today opt to "do it all" simultaneously, and attempt to juggle both motherhood and a career.
But the results can be considerably less than successful. The
moment a working woman is married, her co-workers and
superiors begin to treat her differently, suspicious that she may
commit the sin of childbirth. In view of such attitudes, it is not
surprising that these married women come to fear pregnancy
(no matter how sincerely they may desire it) and are reluctant
to let their bosses know they are pregnant until the last moment
for fear of losing their competitive edge for promotion or
tenure.

Women I have interviewed who are working in business,
education, and medicine were conflicted when they first found
out they were pregnant (and these were planned pregnancies).
Margaret is typical.

"I felt like I would be in trouble if my supervisor found out.
I wanted to have a child, but at the same time I didn't want to
jeopardize my career. I kept it a secret until the end of my fifth
month when I started to show. I almost felt guilty for having
become pregnant. My company only has a two-month maternity leave policy, and I sort of didn't want anybody to be aware
that I was pregnant for any longer than was necessary. I
remember rushing back to work in five weeks just so they would
continue to take me seriously. I guess I didn't want them to
notice that I had given birth."

The story was similar with Carol, a resident in pediatrics at a
metropolitan teaching hospital. When she began crying in the
hallway, I asked her what was wrong. "I don't know why I'm
here," she told me, trying to stop the tears. "I should be home
with my baby. I'm taking care of everybody else's kids, but I'm
afraid to stay home with mine." Carol indicated that a prolonged maternity leave might endanger completion of her

residency. She felt guilty at work, but too frightened to risk her place on the career ladder.

If this fear that compels new mothers to hurry back to work seems excessive, consider the importance attached to a wife's income these days. Quite often, even during the engagement or going-together period, a woman's salary plus her opportunity for advancement are openly taken into account by the man who eventually takes her for his wife. With women liberated from strictly homemaker roles, men no longer have to feel inadequate if their wives share the burden of supporting the family. On the contrary, it is not unusual for a man to quote with pride the earning power of the woman he is marrying. And together, husband and wife plan the road ahead, the future designed to avoid financial inadequacy, by adding in her salary to his, often with no thought given to even the most limited amount of time out for pregnancy or child care.

All this is making it impossible for women to feel adequate. On the one hand, society tells them to pay attention to their biological clocks and not postpone marriage and childbearing beyond the age for safe pregnancy and childbirth. On the other hand, the priority message is that they should be as ambitious and aggressively competitive as men in working toward career advancement. These messages are inherently contradictory.

What we are witnessing is a new attack on femininity, a new form of an old misogynist attitude. It is reminiscent of the attack led by fashion designers and photographers that reduced the ideal woman to a skeleton. In the late 1950s and early 1960s American women did not know whether to laugh or cry as they watched the introduction of dramatically thin models like Twiggy from Europe. To many, such models were little more than a joke. But soon, American models were all Twiggy-thin, and women of normal size felt a desperate need to lose weight. Young girls were demoralized by their own pubescence, especially by the thickening of their thighs and hips. The internal tug-of-war this created spawned an epidemic of anorexia nervosa and other eating disorders that is still with us.

Although some lessons have been learned as a result of this epidemic (skeletal models are no longer used for girls to emulate, but many women are still ashamed of normal levels of body fat), now most media, especially women's magazines, have begun to focus on the new demand: the priority of continued job productivity and the avoidance or limitation of absence due to pregnancy and childbirth. These magazines are influencing and affecting most women to some degree, as did the pressure to be Twiggy-thin, but to what degree women have been affected remains to be seen. Undoubtedly, some women will attempt to ignore the trend and take pride in their pregnancy and time at home, but even for these, economic hard times and society's increasing focus on materialism will make this more and more difficult.

For many college-educated women, the birth of a child appears financially dangerous not only in terms of time away from work but also for the change it will make in the woman's image after she returns to the job. One reflection of this is found in an August 1988 article in the *New York Times*, "Women in the Law Say Path Is Limited by 'Mommy Track,'" which stresses the limitation on women's ability to advance with law firms after childbirth because the women are considered untrustworthy and less committed to the firm as a result of child care or other parental responsibilities. A similar theme was offered in the Diane Keaton film *Baby Boom*. Suddenly presented with a child (an "inheritance" from a British cousin), career woman Keaton's response to the demands of her new charge soon make it impossible for her bosses to take her seriously, and her career goes out the window.

According to this message, women should either skip having children altogether, or keep them a secret, avoiding any mention that might lead management to believe motherhood is causing the woman to give less than 100 percent of her attention to the office job. Imagine the effect this must have on the mother's attitude toward her children and the quality of the time she spends with them!

Help here might come via increased financial support from

business or government for greatly improved day care for working mothers, but so far no such help has been forthcoming under the stewardship of a conservative administration. On the contrary, cutbacks have been the order of the day. And today's woman often fears to be vocal about her wishes in this regard (a fear not shared by her sisters in the 1960s) because it will draw attention to her femininity in the highly competitive marketplace.

Fear of mentioning children during business hours can also be the case for men who find themselves in the primary parent role. A look at the Dustin Hoffman character in *Kramer vs. Kramer* demonstrates how one becomes removed from the "promotional track" and demoted to the "parent track" when business supervisors are made aware of the employee's distraction as a result of his parenting role. In this film, Ted Kramer's wife left him and their son, Billy. Ted becomes the primary parent and tells his boss what happened. His boss then advises him to send Billy to live with relatives because the deal they are working on is all important. A while later the boss expresses his concern about Ted's parent role and ultimately fires him. The lesson is painfully clear. Ted has committed the greatest sin in a competitive corporation: he brought his parenting concerns to the office.

Although some men will find themselves in Ted Kramer's position, it is primarily women who are and will continue to be most sinned against in this regard. The most compliant will simply give up before they begin, deciding that career is everything, leaving no time for marriage and children. But many, perhaps the majority, will find themselves in the middle of the spectrum, nervously becoming pregnant, guiltily going back to work as soon as possible, worried while at work that their children are being inadequately attended to by an indifferent caretaker, and frightened that their career will suffer because they are worried about their children.

Such fear and guilt will contaminate the quality time between mother and child. And here we reach the crux of the matter. The child may perceive Mother's guilt as her being emotionally fragile and feel that he or she needs to be mother's protector. This dynamic will be intensified in families where the father is emotionally unable to provide or express an adequate degree of intimacy, nurturance, and caring for his wife. The child will sense that a caring vacuum exists and will attempt to fill it himself or herself. And this is the fertile ground in which many obsessive-compulsive disorders develop.

In contrast to all this, television sitcoms such as *The Cosby Show* taunt and tantalize children (as well as their mothers and fathers) with the portrayal of parents who, despite demanding careers, appear to find unlimited time to spend with their children, time during which they focus on their children's problems, guiding them about friendships, romances, school-work, ethics, and are unendingly patient and understanding.

These newer family shows have their antecedents in *Ozzie and Harriet, I Remember Mama, Father Knows Best, The Waltons, Leave It to Beaver,* and many others. But what characterized most of the older shows, whether sitcoms or dramas, was the rational behavior of the children. Given appropriate parental behavior, they were good, normal kids. What characterizes *Cosby* and others in this genre is not the normalcy of the kids but the superperceptiveness of the parents and the perfect support, thoughtfulness, and care they give their children.

What must today's real-life child of working parents think when he or she is tantalized by such television superparents? These mothers and fathers help their children in whatever way is needed, working with them or talking to them about the most intimate problems in their lives and with seemingly no time limit! A residue of jealousy, loneliness, and rage must accrue to these young viewers with their noses pressed metaphorically against the television screen, viewing the "goodies" of unlimited nurturing, understanding, and support that cannot be gotten from their own parents who come home from work exhausted and depleted.

And there is still more. These underparented, obsessional charges—these products of two working parents who have left child care in the hands of nannies or governesses or baby-sitters or day care—become aware quite early that, for them, the demand for achievement will be even greater than it was for their mothers and fathers (who were usually raised by their biological parents). Observing their parents' struggle for financial adequacy, these children realize that they too will one day have to engage in such a battle, one which will be greater than that of their parents, a struggle not for success but to avoid being seen as a failure.

The early development of the marketplace, whether in the Middle East or in Andean mountain villages, served to maintain the existence of the family by promoting an exchange of needed goods. In the Age of Obsession, we have a worldwide marketplace that exists solely for itself. It supports financial speculation and greed more than family needs. As individuals and married couples rush into this marketplace to compete, we are seeing an abandonment and subordination of children's emotional needs on a scale not seen since the industrial revolution when children were leased to mines and factories. And it is all in the name of greed. "Greed is good," says the Michael Douglas character in his movie *Wall Street*.

He might have offered a more familiar quotation: "You can't be too rich or too thin." It was in connection with the second half of this maxim that I appeared on *The David Susskind Show* in 1978. Looking at me skeptically, Susskind said, "You're not going to tell me that the fashion industry is responsible for anorexia nervosa?"

"Well," I answered, "I'm not going to say they're *entirely* responsible, but they have certainly turned something that was a rare illness into an epidemic illness."

I had decided to go on Susskind's program as a result of a meeting with Michael Perchek, then head of the Federal Trade Commission. In the course of that meeting, I said to him, "We have to do something about those skinny models and what they're causing women to do. Those magazine covers ought to be labeled, 'This Picture Could Be Hazardous to Your Health.' Can't you bring this danger to the public's attention?"

He smiled at me and said, "*You* do it."

So I set out on a very calculated mission. I could not get a warning published in the women's magazines, but I did appear on talk show after talk show.

It took more than half a decade for the message to penetrate, but it finally happened. One morning I was listening to *Today*, and I heard Jane Pauley ask a fashion designer she was interviewing, "So, are the models this spring going to be *anorexic* again?"

And I said to myself, "Thank God. We are finally going to steer the culture in a different direction." And in the last few years, the models have clearly put on weight.

Now I am saying much the same thing about the culture, but in a larger sense. We have learned some lessons as a result of the epidemic outbreak of anorexia nervosa. We no longer utilize skeletal models for women to emulate. Thus we have begun to get rid of half the "You can't be too rich or too thin" maxim. Now we must try to mediate the "too rich" half as well. We must commit ourselves to changing this nation's obsession with riches in order to stop parents from chasing financial adequacy to the detriment of their children. The cultural machine must be steered in a new direction.

Meanwhile the many individuals whose fate it is to suffer from obsessive-compulsive disorders must be treated. The tools for understanding them and helping them return their lives to normalcy must be used. It is for them and their families, as well as the men and women who will be charged with treating them, that this book is written.

THREE
Familial Origins

Dependency and trust are necessary to enable a child to risk change, tolerate the new, and ultimately develop the character trait of flexibility; in other words, to grow. The parent or parents who foster the development of this dependency and trust are the instruments of the child's safety. What does one need in order to become another's instrument of safety? Energy, confidence, tenderness, generosity, consistency, and, of course, time to offer these to a child.

But if it is these parental attributes that are the key to avoidance of OCD, why is it that the same parents who produce an obsessional child may also produce another (or even several others) without such a disorder?

Every child is constitutionally different, and this is observable from the moment of birth. Parent-child interactions will enhance constitutional strengths and/or exacerbate constitutional vulnerabilities. The child who displays tension in its first weeks, with frequent muscle tensing and intense crying (perhaps simply as a result of problems with the digestive system or another physical condition) may be born to a couple who are themselves confident about their parenting. If they have the tools and time to become the instrument of the child's safety, or if they have a strong, supportive extended family or even very capable help at home, they will probably be able to mediate the child's constitutional tension. But if this same child should be born into an already anxious home, his own sensitivity may further weaken parental coping ability. Crying may be experienced as a reflection of parental inadequacy by either parent, and a tense, anxiety-exacerbating relationship may be formed with the parents.

A child who perceives a parent in distress due to spousal or health problems experiences an absence of confidence in that parent's ability to take care of him and make him safe and secure. Very often, such a child perceives that his own safety can only be improved by efforts to make the parents less distressed. The first way the child may do this is to minimize his own needs, thus placing fewer demands for care on the distressed parent. This leads the child to fear his own needs and to see them as dangerous to his parent's well-being, and therefore perilous to himself. The relationship formed between this child and parent fails to enable the child to develop a basic, healthy dependency. No longer a safe person for the child to depend upon, the parent has become, instead, only a symbol of dependency. Whatever strength that parent has—whatever strength he or she is able to give the child—is now experienced as the child's creation. And the child secretly takes responsibility for the maintenance of that strength. An implicit reversal of dependency has developed between parent and child without either of them acknowledging it or even recognizing it consciously.

For the child, the most dangerous problem with this is that it deflects care that might be (or should be) offered to him. He makes someone else the focus, disallowing his own needs. He becomes instrumental in creating a deficit of direct parental identity messages. Since his parent (or parents) may indeed be exhausted and depleted as a result of responsibilities, obligations, or health, money, and even chronic emotional problems, the child's offer of (and skill at providing) emotional help tempts parents into acceptance. As this process evolves, parents and child form a relationship where they collude in an implicit reversal of dependency that will leave the child feeling angry, deprived, unfocused upon, liked only for his ability to service others, and empty of a sense of identity.

The father in these families is usually experienced by the wife as emotionally inaccessible or detached, focused on issues and people outside the family. He is not someone who allows for intimacy between his wife and himself, and his relationship with his children is no closer. There are many possible reasons for his emotional distance from his wife: conflicts in his family or origin, or personality and mood disorders. He often appears to function successfully in a work or career environment that makes no demands for personal intimacy but only for achievement. His wife then functions within the family as an emotionally abandoned person with many unmet needs; and together, mother and father create the environment for their child's development of OCD.

Lara is such an example. She was described by her mother as unhappy from birth, and difficult to calm when she was an infant. Lara resisted holding and being carried. Such efforts at pampering simply made her cry more intensely with increased agitation. Her mother was unprepared for this temperament, especially since Lara's older brother had been playful and relaxed since infancy. At the time of Lara's birth, her father was transferred to another city by his company, and it was decided that the family would temporarily remain behind in their small apartment. Lara remembers (with extraordinary clarity) her early childhood years of frightening insecurity. She experienced her mother as unhappy and perhaps "on the verge of leaving."

Lara explains, "I was always frightened in that horrible apartment. I just hated everything there—the neighborhood, just everything. I'm sure my mother hated me and the apartment. When I have panic attacks now, I feel like I did back then. I feel like I could get sent back there."

Lara became a help to her mother at an early age, as well as her mother's constant companion. She helped around the house, in the kitchen, and kept her mother company when she went to the market or visited Lara's grandmother in a convalescent home each day. Lara never felt proud of herself. She felt as if she were just treading water to keep her mother from leaving her. "I just did what I had to, to make my mother's life bearable . . . so she wouldn't leave us."

By the time Lara was seven, the family's finances had improved and they were settled in a large house in a fashionable suburb. Pressures on Lara's father to move up on the corporate ladder kept him at work for very long hours on a regular basis, so that even though the family were reunited in their big house, Lara's mother was still responsible for the emotional work of raising the children. Although she ran the home virtually alone, her husband maintained the attitude that she was a childish, temperamental woman who could not understand the demands made on him by the world of work—the only real world, insofar as he was concerned. As the years of suburban life went on, a family pattern became established: father a high-strung, seldom home workaholic; older brother an athletic, casual teen with many friends; and Lara, a precocious and articulate companion to her mother, happier around her mother's friends than her own peers.

Lara came to therapy at the age of twelve with diagnoses of obsessive-compulsive disorder, anorexia nervosa, panic disorder, and multiple phobias. She was four feet ten and fifty-eight pounds (normal weight would have been eighty-five). She was petite, spoke in a small voice, and continuously fidgeted with her rings and many bracelets. She seemed to be counting them over and over. She touched her fingertips with her thumbs repeatedly as if counting them as well. As she became more tense, her ritualistic behavior sped up. It seemed as if she were in a race as she frantically repeated her rituals. She parted and reparted her hair with her fingers, and she added additional behaviors as the session progressed.

Although Lara's anorexia responded to treatment fairly early, the symptoms that persisted well into the third year of therapy were her more basic obsessive-compulsive behaviors. While they diminished in frequency and intensity, they were clearly the core symptoms with which she protected herself from feelings of distress. They warded off either focused fears of real or imagined consequence (such as her mother not returning, or all her schoolmates shunning her), or controlled painful levels of anxiety and unwelcome energy by the rapid repetition of safe-making activities. As Lara raced through counting her rings, rotating them on her fingers, and methodically rearranging the spacing of her bracelets, she was soothing herself.

She had always suffered from excessive anxiety, and this anxiety was clearly a response to real situations in her life: her fears of going back to the run-down neighborhood, an awareness about her mother's stress, and her father's emotional distance. It became important to Lara not to depend upon her parents, but at the same time she seemed to cling to them for at least their physical proximity. If her mother was nearby, she was safe. But it was not her mother who made her feel safe; it was the ritual of keeping her mother nearby that produced the security. (Obsessional individuals often experience ambivalent feelings toward the parent on whom they depend the most. Since they resent having to depend on anyone besides themselves, it is a hostile dependency, thus the ambivalence.)

If Lara remains in this state of mistrust, she will develop a host of rituals to create a tentative sense of calm that will partially alleviate her feelings of anxiety and depression. Since the mechanism only partially succeeds, its employment is constantly increased in the hope that it will finally provide a state of emotional security. The mechanism of inventing a danger and then figuring out a ritual behavior as the solution to the danger attributes power to the ritual and results in a sense of grandiose control in its user.

In essence, Lara was inventing her own superstitions (as other OCDs do), creating a closed system in much the same way rules and rituals are created for primitive religions. And like those religions, Lara's superstitions told her when to feel guilty, virtuous, frightened, or secure. By trusting in such a religion, one becomes responsible for maintaining its values by obeying the rules and following the rituals. Failing to do so produces pain (criticism and fear), while successful compliance produces pride and a sense of security.

Lara believed that her rituals kept her mother safe. On a metaphysical level, she believed that she was her mother's keeper and, thus, the keeper of herself as well.

Lara's childhood memories of anxiety and depression indicate a constitutional vulnerability to obsessive-compulsive disorder. Her awareness of these uncomfortable feelings plus a lack of positive parental identity messages have had a profound effect on her self-esteem over the developmental years. She regarded herself as unlikable and repelling, and this became a theme in many therapy sessions: "I'm just a miserable person. I'm ugly, unlikable, stupid, and boring. I've always been miserable, since I was born. I don't think that anybody ever liked me and I don't see why anybody should."

This sort of self-reference is typical of Lara when she talks about herself, but when reality testing is done, she resists.

I might ask her, "Do others react to you in a way that verifies your negative feelings? Do they turn away while you're talking? Do they make faces at you to indicate that they don't like you? Do they call you any of the names that you call yourself?"

She responded with, "I don't know."

I pursued the testing: "You aren't confronting your feelings about this; why not?"

"You don't understand. I can't confront my feelings about

this. Maybe you'll never understand. It's like a ritual to think about myself this way. I just do. And I can't examine it."

Such low self-esteem is often characteristic of those suffering from obsessive-compulsive disorders and is generally the result of poor parental identity messages, those statements one hears from parents that when combined form a sense of self. These identity messages may also take the form of parental postures, attitudes, and conceptions by the child. All children receive a variety of these messages about themselves from their parents: "You are cute, smart, clever, sweet, thoughtful, handsome, pretty, strong, interesting (inferred), assertive, stubborn, fresh, stupid, boring (inferred), homely (inferred), inattentive, have good taste, have bad taste," and so on.

The reason that "interesting," "boring," and "homely" are designated "inferred" is that they are rarely stated to a child but are rather *inferred* by the child. They are inferred, in the case of "boring," as a result of an absence of focus, attention, or eye contact by parents. In the case of "interesting," the inference is made from the frequency of focus, attention, and eye contact as well as by the parents remembering the child's activities, achievements, and likes and dislikes (this may be with regard to food, clothing, or preferred games). "Homely" is the inference children can make when they are never told they are attractive, handsome, or pretty.

Inferred parental identity messages are usually negative (with the exception of "interesting") and these ideas result from the absence of positive comments. If a girl such as Lara is never told she is pretty, she will assume she is ugly. She will not have the ego strength to believe that she really *is* pretty, only her parents forgot to tell her so. If a child is never told she is smart, she will infer that she is stupid. If a child is always spoken to by a parent on the run, over-the-shoulder, with little eye contact, the child will infer that she is boring or unimportant.

When a child experiences a lack of direct parental identity messages (praises, comments, and criticisms) and has accumulated a large store of inferred negative messages, the child perceives herself as empty. The child who has had to do the work of inferring who he or she is also has developed a persistent internal critical voice to compensate for the lack of a positive external parental voice. The dominance of inferred negative parental messages, combined with the mechanism of inferring instead of incorporating, fosters mistrust instead of trust and isolation instead of intimacy* in a meaningful sense. The result is a phenomenon that might be called developmental emptiness. This condition is revealed when the patient makes such statements as:

> "I feel like a fraud."
> "I feel like nobody."
> "I am nothing."
> "I feel like there's nobody inside."
> "When I try to think about myself I get numb, like I'm looking for something that isn't there."
> "I just try to be like whoever I'm with at the time."

When a child suffers from developmental emptiness and utilizes obsessional defenses to cope with the accompanying anxiety and depression, that primary emptiness becomes compounded by social separation. This happens because instead of creating friendships, the child is preoccupied with behavioral self-control. The resulting social vacuum enhances the negative inferring mechanism within the individual so that he or she resorts to mistrust and isolation, spiraling deeper into emptiness as the mechanisms of obsessional thinking and obsessive-compulsive defenses dominate.

Fortunately, Lara responded well to treatment. As mentioned previously, her anorexia symptoms decreased during the first year, in part because she was amenable to my suggestion of assertive refeeding and meal supervision by her mother. Although there were several minor recurrences of the anorexia, they appeared to be a form of acting out on Lara's part

*These useful paired concepts were first presented by Erik Erikson in *Childhood and Society* (New York: W. W. Norton, 1950), chapter 7.

rather than a compelling obsessional drive to become thinner. In each instance her mother's strong stand brought the recurrences under control.

As for Lara's underlying obsessive-compulsive symptoms, these required a far longer period of treatment, a continuous schedule of therapy sessions that eventually filled her emptiness, allowing her gradually to give up her many self-soothing rituals and live a normal life.

While Lara might have to contend with higher than average levels of anxiety, she is luckier than most sufferers of OCD in that she became ritual-free.

FOUR

When OCD Begins

ANNABELLE: "I feel like it was always there."

DIANE: "I didn't have any of this until after the accident."

KATHARINE: "It happened when I came out of the hospital, at sixteen."

DEBBIE: "I've been like this since I was six."

NINA: "It happened with anorexia."

BETH: "It started at nine, right after he started molesting me."

MARTHA: "I've been like this since the sixth grade."

LORETTA: "I've been trying to stay clean enough since my father did things to me at five."

In the obsessive-compulsive individual, the seeds of vulnerability may be sown during the first four years of life, for it is during this period of time that bonding between mother and child takes place. The seeds may also precede birth, in the form of a constitutional (hereditary) predisposition to anxiety and/or depression. But even when both of these factors, heredity and family dynamics, are present, OCD symptoms often await a trauma before emerging. This trauma may be as subtle as the social demands of adolescence or as catastrophic as child molestation.

For Katharine (mentioned earlier as buying an answering machine because her rituals left no time for talking with friends), it was her hospitalization. Prior to this, she had undergone a series of tragedies: the suicide of her father when she was fourteen; the death of her governess, her primary caretaker, when she was sixteen; and shortly after that, the onset of anorexia nervosa. Even with all this, it was only after what she experienced as traumatic, insensitive psychiatric hospitalization—six months "locked up" in what she describes as an "isolating and humiliating experience"—that she came home, retreated from friends and family, and developed an array of obsessive-compulsive rituals vast enough to occupy her every waking moment.

Her history suggests that the ritualistic nature of anorexia nervosa simply led her beyond eating-related behaviors into cleanliness, organizing, and arranging behaviors. She often reflected back on times in her early teens when she had felt no need for any of these behaviors, and she is puzzled by the onset of her eating disorder and the OCD rituals at the age of sixteen. She views the hospitalization as "the straw that broke the camel's back."

For Diane, the trauma was much more subtle. Although hospitalization (a severe accident at age sixteen) was also involved, the onset of her obsessional behavior did not occur until several years afterward. Diane remembers her social and family life as normal prior to her accident (which left her in a coma for nine days and did much short-term neurological damage), not at all characterized by either rigidity or compulsivity. And this sense of normalcy continued for nearly three years after the accident, until the completion of her follow-up surgeries.

At that point, the end of her first year in college, "Things began to fall apart." Why? It appears that once her recovery was complete, after having maintained the heroic attitude that characterized all her behavior in the face of painful surgery and painful psychotherapy, all she was left with was a scarred breast and a permanently injured shoulder and arm. She then retreated into obsessive-compulsive behavior because that post-recovery period, despite its apparent lack of drama, was the time of her deepest despair. She felt that she should have been capable of independence, but in truth, she was not, and her sense of shame about this made it impossible for her to turn to her parents.

In contrast, Annabelle remembers her early childhood and her relationship with her mother as always full of conflict and fear. She has no recollection of any trauma or time period that brought on her OCD symptoms, for she employed rituals for security as far back as she can remember in the hope that they would make her mother friendly to her and stop her mother from "freezing her out."

Debbie also can not remember a time before she resorted to rituals, but her mother recalls, "Debbie just stopped at six." This was immediately after the nanny, who had been the child's primary caretaker, left without notice or preparation.

Nina became ill with anorexia at twelve, then withdrew into a psychologically caused inability to speak, as well as rituals of organizing and cleanliness during every waking moment. She had to be hospitalized. Puberty is the most likely precipitant of her anorexia nervosa, and it is common to see either a simultaneous onset of OCD rituals or a rapid subsequent development of them when an individual develops anorexia.

With Beth there was no question about the trauma that produced OCD. It was molestation. The last of four children, she was left without a father at age five (he deserted the family). Her mother managed a bar and was an alcoholic. Her brothers and sister, considerably older than Beth, moved out a year after the father deserted. Beth became a latch-key child, nearly always home alone. A next-door neighbor, a man in his thirties, gave her an occasional pat on the head and a smile. At the age of nine, she was invited to his apartment. He explained to her that if she wanted to be his friend, she had to have intercourse with him. Crying and bleeding, she discovered that this was an extremely painful experience. Like other molesters of children, the neighbor told her not to tell anyone else. He also told her that if she wanted to see him again, they would have to repeat this experience. Beth describes him as affectionate through all this, and it was the first closeness that she recalled receiving from anyone. She decided that the attention was worth the pain. From the age of nine to the age of twelve, she was, in effect, his lover. She was terrified about what she was doing and assumed, in her own mind, complete responsibility for it. From the beginning of this relationship, she began to shower frequently each day. She soon added handwashing and rituals of superstition.

Her first emotional defense in coping with this overwhelming experience was to develop obsessive-compulsive behaviors. Her fear and daily dread of these experiences made her wish that she could talk to someone about them, but the guilt and sense of wrongdoing she felt made talking to anyone out of the question. Her acceptance of these horrendous conditions for having a relationship with another person is indicative of how desperate she was for some kind of attachment: even this was better than nothing. When Beth was thirteen, the man said he did not want to see her anymore. She had, by then, adjusted to the conditions of the relationship, and she was heartbroken and felt abandoned. She despaired of ever having a caring relationship. After that, she ritualized most of her daily behavior and finally entered treatment at age twenty-five.

Molestation was also the trauma that caused the onset of OCD for Loretta. At age five, she was molested by her father. She remembers feeling frightened and repulsed by his behavior. She also remembers that her feelings of security and safety within her family were severely diminished. She no longer felt that her mother would or could protect her from harm.

Despite what appeared to be a normal childhood, Loretta's sense of danger would rarely leave her. She did well in school, succeeded in athletic competition, participated in all the benefits that come from an affluent family—and always felt ashamed that she could not feel good about life.

Her family was impatient with her about the extraordinary amount of time she needed in the bathroom and especially in the shower. She describes cleaning her ears, nose, and the corners of her eyes with cotton swabs dipped in alcohol. She had been told by physicians that this kind of cleaning could be damaging, but her need to clean herself overrode these realistic considerations. Her cleaning here was really her attempt at decontaminating her body.

Girls who are molested in childhood often experience contamination trauma. During child molestation, the child's body is penetrated against her will. The physical act is unwanted and terrifying, and offers proof that she is unprotected in the most profound sense. Her ability to trust and depend upon others is severely damaged. Her need to clean out the contamination to reestablish a sense of physical integrity and safety becomes satisfied by using obsessive-compulsive cleanliness rituals. Since these rituals do not really protect her against the event of molestation or prevent it from recurring, she settles for the symbolic act of the cleaning to compensate her for the violation she has experienced.

On some level, she understands that there is little compensation or protection in her rituals. This understanding requires her to repeat the rituals with increasing, insatiable frequency in order to regulate her fear, which becomes experienced as nonspecific anxiety. She needs to block out the painful idea of being molested.

The most extreme and distressing example of this that I have ever encountered was an eleven-year-old girl who was referred to me for an evaluation of her "atypical anorexia." She had reduced her food intake after what was described as an experience of molestation and rape that lasted twelve hours.

She answered questions politely during our interview but I noticed she continued to spit throughout the meeting. It was clear to me that she was "spitting out semen" in her attempt to "decontaminate" herself. I referred her to a woman psycho-therapist. I told her that I did not think it was fair for her to have to discuss this with a man. The patient was referred for therapy within weeks of the event and made a good connection with her new therapist.

In the cases of Beth and Loretta, fifteen years had elapsed before they were able to talk about these experiences and the feelings they engendered. During those fifteen years, their decontaminating behaviors became part of their system for regulating their anxiety. Both of their lives had become ritual ridden due to the childhood trauma of sexual molestation.

The traumatic events that led to the onset of Martha's obsessive-compulsive behavior were far less obvious than those for Beth and Loretta. Martha describes a happy childhood with lots of success in school, both academically and socially, until the sixth grade and adolescence. At that time, she recalls getting the message from her mother that social life was not particularly important and that grades were the priority.

So impressed was Martha by this message that she felt compelled to give up her place as one of the popular kids and buckle down full-time to studying. She quickly rose to the top of her class in achievement, graduating as valedictorian, but she experienced the rest of her schooling as less fun and became socially withdrawn. It was during her initial social withdrawal that she began looking for something that would feel as good as her childhood success (socially as well as academically). She decided that it should be eating. When she ate pasta, it was one noodle at a time, taking two hours. She also became preoccupied with elimination, especially the time of day it occurred, and this dominated her daytime schedule.

By the time Martha entered treatment (in her early twenties), she had amassed a record of academic excellence, but no social relationships and, after college, an existence so reclusive that it did not include employment. Years before Martha had inferred from her mother's warning about excessive socializing that she should make radical changes in her life. Clearly, a great lack of communication had to exist between Martha and her mother to allow Martha to come to such a point of withdrawal, a process dangerous to Martha in that it invited her to fill the vacuum created by her lost social life with self-satisfying behaviors.

All of this occurred at the beginning of what should have been her adolescence, socially as well as physically. There was clearly a vagueness as to cause other than the simultaneous fear of adolescence and of failing in the future (academically and vocationally), and an inability on Martha's part to use her relationship with her parents to discuss her fears.

The beginnings of obsessive-compulsive symptoms in the eight people mentioned here ranged from five to sixteen years of age. The reasons for their beginnings varied from the subtle need to become an adolescent, to the experience of being damaged at the hands of others. What all of these reasons have in common is that in some way each person had to cope with a situation that was not a one-time event but continued in life, was terrifying, and could not be discussed with parents. Lines of dependency either did not exist or were disrupted by the nature of the crisis.

In the case of Annabelle and Debbie, lines of dependency never developed. In the case of Loretta, her father's acts against her made her feel separate from her family at the age of five, and unable to depend upon them. Nina and Katharine were separated from their parents by hospitalization. However fragile their lines of dependency prior to the hospitalization, it was this experience that seems to have severed the lines completely. In some cases, these lines can be rebuilt on parents' initiative; in others, they cannot.

In Beth's case, her attempt to develop a dependency with a person outside the family to compensate for the absence of any with her mother resulted in severe molestation that she tolerated in the hope that she could form a real dependency in her victimizer. That dependency produced nothing but pain for her, and she withdrew into rituals. Diane's lines of dependency were severed by her shame about still finding herself in emotional need after all the assistance her parents had given her following an accident.

The date at which an individual develops obsessive-compulsive behavior is often difficult to pinpoint. Since most rituals can be kept secret from parents for years, we often have only the self-reporting of the patient to guide us, and this can be misleading. We do know that OCD is not an adolescent behavior. It begins earlier. Most of the people I see, especially girls, report the onset of rituals at the age of nine or ten. But others have reported children exhibiting this behavior at ages six, seven, and eight.

The age at which the behavior begins may indicate the point at which that person experienced despair about being able to trust or depend upon important persons in her life. The despair over lost dependency provokes the withdrawal and turning inward toward self-reassurance in the form of repetitious rituals. In the cases mentioned here, different elements of each person's life brought her to the conclusion that no one was there for her, and each was frightened enough to need to constantly regulate the resulting anxiety.

The question arises: Would they have developed OCD behavior if these events had not occurred? Probably not, but the lack of dependency would have remained, ready to provoke OCD behavior should other such events occur. And that leads to a second question: Why did these events cause OCD as opposed to some other stress-oriented responses, such as panic disorder, phobias, or psychosomatic illnesses, for instance?"

The answer lies again in lack of dependency and in the sense of despair that characterizes those individuals who have been denied a strong, guiding relationship with a parent figure. Confront such individuals with great emotional distress, and OCD defenses may well be called into play. Nowhere is this connection made clearer than in the case of OCD sufferers whose childhood was affected by parental alcoholism.

CHILDREN OF ALCOHOLICS

Because alcoholism so seriously impairs one parent and thereby depletes the other, it creates a tremendous nurturance vacuum within the family, and the child tries to compensate by filling the vacuum with her own comforting. Her personality is often the foil (or complement) to the alcoholic parent. Where the father is the alcoholic, the daughter becomes the compensatory personality. From her perspective, he is irresponsible toward the rest of the family, especially his wife. Threatened by the instability, the child tries to make it up to mother, to give her the missing support. If the daughter can strengthen the mother, the daughter will also be making herself more secure.

The daughter's obsessionality or overthinking begins to develop as she attempts to take care of her mother (and sometimes her father, too). She is left to turn inward to meet her own needs, turning to rituals in order to create a sense of parenting that she cannot get from this depleted couple. Although she loves them, she will have hostile feelings that she will struggle to repress.

She is always contemptuous of her parents, as she regards their strength as fraudulent. She is angry at the weakness in the spousal support system, fearful that it may collapse, and she will then experience abandonment. If her mother is an alcoholic, the daughter must work even harder to keep that parent stable so that she can pretend that the woman is healthy. In effect, she is mothering her mother and pretending to be the recipient of the nurturance she, herself, is generating.

This process of the child's generating nurturance and denying that it originated with herself requires much self-reassuring behavior. Personal superstitions are brought into play as self-created parental messages from an imaginary, strong parent. The requirement for this self-reassurance is endless, since it is spurious. Overthinking about details, perfectionism, rigidity, and obsessive-compulsive rituals become the tools or defenses that buttress the child's pretending that she has secure parents and, therefore, a secure self.

Alcoholism within the family becomes the factor that disables a parent from being healthy enough to adequately nurture a child. The child of the alcoholic develops an obsessional system to cope with the nurturance drain that the alcoholism has created. Lauren is an example. Of her relationship with her alcoholic father, she says, "He's more married to the bottle than to my mother. I always feel like he's my responsibility, and when he's drunk, he says he's closer to me than anyone else. I hate it, but on the other hand, I fear losing this weird connection to him."

Twenty-six years old when she entered treatment, Lauren was a resident in psychiatry at a metropolitan teaching hospital. She felt overwhelmed with obsessive-compulsive thoughts and behaviors. Her day was one of endless rituals. She had taken one year off between her internship and residency and had developed a reclusive lifestyle, seeing only members of her immediate family: her parents, who were debating the merits of divorcing each other; her younger sister, who was doing well in graduate school; and her accident-prone, drug-involved brother (also younger), who had been arrested for serious traffic violations.

When asked about her relationships with members of her family other than her father, she indicated, "I feel as if they would all like to divorce *me*. My sister's always annoyed with me. She's begun to act as if she's older than me. My brother always sounds distracted when he's talking to me, as if he can't wait for the conversation to be over. My mother still calls me for advice, but she's totally unwilling to work on their marriage. So it's a mess."

In discussing the possibility of divorce for her parents, Lauren said, "I'm more worried about my dad than my mom, but I still feel like I have to take care of both of them. Each one is afraid that I'll love the other more, so I have to continually reassure them that neither is in danger of being abandoned by me. In a way, I'm more their parent than ever."

"How does meeting their needs make you feel?" I asked.

"It upsets me . . . you know that."

"What if you gave up the role of reassurer?"

"I would be panicked."

Lauren felt that she had always suffered from extraordinary anxiety. She believed that it had come about in reaction to her family system, but the intensity of that anxiety and panic might have been much less severe had she been blessed with a less vulnerable nervous system. Since her anxiety was intolerable most of the time, her need to regulate with OCD rituals and excessive exercise was intense and nearly constant.

During Lauren's first weeks of treatment, she mysteriously referred to the possibility of "losing it completely" if she were not able to contain her level of stress. I repeatedly tried to get her to clarify what she meant by "losing it," but she would not, although she continued to make references to being out of control.

One day she came into the office looking pale and was unable to sit down. She walked back and forth across the room and, after several self-interrupted, incomplete sentences, she glared at me and announced, "I've lost it completely."

I asked, "What does that mean?"

"It means that all of my rituals didn't work this time."

"And?"

"And . . ." She looked down at the floor. ". . . I'm the same as the patients in my locked unit. I cut myself. I know what that means. It means I'm pretty sick."

"Is this what you meant by 'losing it completely'?"

"Yes. I did this when I was a teenager. I was seeing a psychiatrist then, and he told me that if I didn't stop, he would have me locked up for a long time. So I didn't tell him about it anymore. I acted so healthy that I was excused from seeing him anymore."

Those knowing Lauren only in her professional capacity would have been amazed to discover the existence of her OCD.

Her facade was impeccable. She was always tastefully dressed in a New England, conservative fashion. Her social manner was genial, engaging, and supportive, in sharp contrast to her inner turmoil and self-mutilating behavior.

Talking about her role as a psychiatric resident, she asked, "How do you think I feel sitting there listening to lectures about self-mutilation, and all the while I'm hoping that no one ever sees my wrists? I have over a dozen scars on each arm. So I nod whenever a patient who cuts herself is presented, feeling like a thief or surely a fraud inside. I don't want to leave psychiatry. I want to beat this problem."

"What makes you cut yourself?"

"Most of the time, all the other stuff—you know, the rituals and the exercises—they use up enough energy so that this doesn't have to happen. It hasn't happened for ten years. I don't want to go back to feeling like that again!"

"But what do you get from cutting yourself?"

"Pain."

"What does the pain do for you?"

"It brings me back."

"It brings you back from what—or where?"

Lauren looked impatient, not so much with me, but with her own difficulty of being the patient. She was more comfortable with the caretaker's role. She continued, "It brings you back from being away from yourself. It's—you know—a dissociative state—" She suddenly interrupted herself, and said with a rapid speech pattern, "I can't believe that I'm talking about myself this way. I just can't believe it." She shook her head. "Anyhow, what I was saying is, I start to feel like I'm going to lose myself. There's no other way I can explain it. I feel myself drifting away from myself, and the pain brings me back."

I suggested that she take time off, but she refused.

"Hard work is all that keeps me going," she insisted. "Anyhow, what if my hospital found out how screwed up I am?"

In truth, Lauren was an exemplary clinician in her hospital

position, and with the exception of two days at the height of her crisis (for which she called in sick), she managed to carry on successfully.

Due to an alcoholic father and a needy mother, Lauren had learned to distrust her parents at an early age. Her previous experience as a patient in psychotherapy reinforced that mistrust. For her, the most difficult obstacle to successful psychotherapy was fear of dependence. Because she saw her parents as needy, her sense of identity was founded on being the care provider (Lauren the psychiatrist) not the receiver of care (Lauren the patient). I could see Lauren's conflict about being a patient in every therapy session. When she responded with straightforward answers that were not sarcastic or self-mocking, she immediately experienced anxiety and retreated to the distancing posture. Despite the well-entrenched nature of this distancing, Lauren managed to give it up after only a year in treatment.

Claudia, also the daughter of an alcoholic father, had vivid recollections of unhealthy family development. She remembered overhearing her aunt say to her mother, "The trouble with you, Marge, is that you went straight from your mother to your daughter [Claudia], without ever growing up." Claudia was eight years old when she overheard this fragment of a conversation.

Like Lauren, Claudia always felt that *she* was the nurturer of her parents. By the age of eight, she was already making important decisions for the family. She routinely decided upon the restaurants they would eat at, the private schools that she and her two younger brothers would attend, and the summer cottages that the family would rent.

Perhaps her parents felt that they were being democratic in offering these choices to their oldest child at such a young age. They might have believed that Claudia would become a better decision maker as an adult because of it. Most likely, however, the decisions were left to Claudia due to her father's drinking. At thirteen, Claudia was hospitalized for what was described as a drug-induced nervous breakdown. She remembered feeling as if she had lost control of her thoughts completely. She also recalled that the most painful part of being in a hospital was being a patient. She had always seen herself as the person in charge or "everyone's caretaker."

She experienced the hospitalization as a humiliating demotion and punishment for failing to continue to take care of her family. She left the hospital after a year, determined never to make that mistake again. She behaved in an exemplary manner throughout high school and college. She resumed her nurturing role as decision maker for her mother, baby-sitter for her brothers, and nursemaid to her father when he was drunk. During her teen years, she even filled her mother's place as her father's companion and confidante.

Claudia became increasingly anxious as she assumed the responsibility for keeping her brothers in school and acting as a buffer between her parents. Unlike many children who simply fantasize exorbitant responsibility for their family's well-being and marriage cohesion, Claudia was the central nurturing figure and organizational head of the family.

Within one year of graduating college, Claudia's compulsive behavior, especially her neatness, rigidity, and exercising, had many of her friends worried. Then she began to drink. After experiencing blackouts, she entered therapy at age twenty-two. Her immediate problem was her fear of a breakdown like the one she had experienced at the age of thirteen. She felt that her obsessive-compulsive behaviors were unbearable, and that her anxiety was breaking through, no matter how much she busied herself with rituals. She held a responsible job and feared becoming observably weird there.

Claudia reported that her friends, whose confidante she had been, complained that they found her secretive. Although she was always there with "a shoulder to cry on" (just as she had been with her parents), her friends felt Claudia never broke down and expressed her own inner feelings. Claudia agreed. She realized she was inaccessible to others, and she hated it. When I asked if she thought that she could become accessible, Claudia replied with a shrug of the shoulders. "I hope so, but I really don't know."

"How do you hope that therapy can help you?"

"I don't know. I'm not sure why I'm here. I've read a lot of the literature on children of alcoholics, and I know I fit the pattern. I seek relationships with abusive men. Nice men turn me off. I have a hard time confronting people, and I put up with all sorts of requests for favors I don't want to do. I'm always worried about what others think of me. I never feel like I'm doing a good-enough job. The list just goes on and on. I don't know how you can help me since I'm aware of what's going on. I have most of the insights. I guess I'm hoping that you'll do something to make these insights work." She smiled nervously, with a slight laugh. "You're the shrink, and I hope you know something I don't so this will *all go away.*" She said the last words like a mother reassuring her child.

Claudia presented herself as a nonhostile, friendly patient, but this disguised the intensity of her deeply imbedded need to resist the help offered her in therapy. While she had a wish that another person could help her, she had the need to remain in control of the relationship and to parent the therapist. Within her social relationships, she either parented or was abused. Helping her work through this resistance and keeping her in treatment without gratifying either of these needs was the first major step in therapy. She expected the therapist to become one of the two facets of her alcoholic father: abusive or needy. Constant attention must be given to this transference when doing therapy with a patient like Claudia (whom we will meet again—and Lauren also—in chapter 13, "Turning Points").

Alcoholism often produces such destructive behavior, including inconsistency, abuse, incompetence, and failure to communicate, that it creates what could be called a family-nurturance drain. Other problems also produce this situation, although not always in such a clear-cut way. If, for example, one family member suffers from heart trouble or perhaps chronic depression, the resulting focus on this problem may cause other family members to be so depleted that they are incapable of providing adequate nurturance for the growing children. These children then become the self-caretakers and self-soothers who are potential victims of OCD.

FIVE

Eating Disorders

In the years following publication of my book *Treating and Overcoming Anorexia Nervosa,* I have been contacted by many individuals who were desirous of my help and yet not certain they should be calling. Having read the book, they recognized themselves in most of the conduct that characterized the patients—inflexibility, difficulty in making decisions, compulsiveness about daily routines, inability to feel close to others yet good at nurturing them, and suffering continuously from feelings of emptiness—but they were hesitant to phone me for help because they did *not* suffer from anorexia!

The answer to their dilemma was relatively simple. They saw themselves having the more basic personality traits of anorexic patients: difficulty with dependency and trust, traits (and their causes) that are the same whether one's particular defense is compulsive handwashing or anorexia. A lack of proper nurturance produces a need for reassurance and, eventually, a sense of emptiness that the individual struggles to fill with some sort of reassuring conduct (rituals). Since sucking, our earliest method for achieving reassurance, includes food as well as repetition, it is not surprising that many nurture-starved individuals seek reassurance in food-related rituals, while others do so in rituals such as handwashing where no food is directly involved but there is repetition. At the same time, it is not surprising to find individuals who eventually suffer from both such disorders.

Some characteristics of the obsessional personality, particularly the inflexibility and sense of emptiness, can best be understood by examining them as they relate to eating disorders. For example, when anorexia caught the public's attention in the mid-1970s, the generalization that stuck concerned inflexibility and the issue of control. It has been widely stated that anorexics, as they adhere to their routines, are attempting to control their feelings by mastering their bodies, and their bodies' food intake, digestive and elimination functions, weight, and appearance. Let us examine this control issue as it relates to the wider spectrum of obsessional disorders.

When parents of anorexic girls discuss their daughter's preanorexic personality, they use words like "well-behaved," "compliant," "high-achieving," "perfectionist," "rigid," "pleasant," and "well-adjusted." But when they discuss the personality changes wrought by the illness, they delete well-behaved, compliant, pleasant, and well-adjusted and see an intensification of rigidity and perfectionism. They also note new behaviors that are exhibited in defense of the control system that governs their daughter's illness. These new behaviors and traits include defiance, especially when family members attempt to increase the anorexic's caloric intake, reduce her exercise, or restrict the use of laxatives or diuretics. Whether her behavior is overtly confrontational and argumentative or covertly oppositional and manipulative, the anorexic's struggle to prevent others from interfering with her system of control is characterized by an assertiveness, aggression, and defiance not seen previously in her personality.

A moral, ethical, and aesthetic withdrawal occurs at the same time, for the anorexic will resort to any means to maintain her system of control. She no longer shares society's concept of an attractive and healthy appearance with regard to herself. She has departed from group values and withdraws to her obsessional system for emotional safety. Yet throughout all these changes, she remains a nurturer of friends and family.

Unlike non-eating-disordered obsessive-compulsive behavior, anorexia nervosa rewards its victim's superstitious behavior with tangible results. Most obviously, she loses weight. And here the therapist must be careful not to confuse cause and effect. Excessively low weight produces organic mental changes such as depression, withdrawal, anxiety, and a preoccupation with food. But this is a consequence of anorexia, not its cause. For an individual to develop this disease, a flawed child-parent bond was waiting to be tested. There are many possible circumstances that might account for the insufficient dependency, trust, and intimacy within the relationship.

Often an inappropriate degree of nurturing behavior (by the patient) is an important clue. If this is focused on the parents, we can deduce that the patient is filling a caring vacuum. She has perceived exhaustion and depletion on the part of her parents, and, early on, she reversed the flow of dependency so that she has a dominant position in the family and may even maintain her role by encouraging her parents to be emotionally dependent upon her. At the same time, she may play a supportive role with her friends, becoming a "shoulder to cry on."

Unlike most obsessional disorders, anorexia nervosa is conspicious by its victim's changing appearance and eating behavior. Other OCDs can develop undetected for years or be passed off as eccentric but essentially harmless. In addition to offering tangible physical changes as rewards for superstitious behavior, anorexia nervosa is a form of OCD where malnutrition creates an organic mind syndrome that enhances obsessionality and offers its victim the secondary gain of assertiveness and aggression as she defeats those in her environment who mobilize in opposition to her disordered behavior. Ultimately, the style of her struggle with others—her disfigured appearance, ascetic willpower in depriving herself of nutrition, special thinness, eating rituals—will all coalesce to form a pseudofunctional identity that will alleviate her terrifying sense of emptiness.

The development of anorexia nervosa usually occurs at some imminent point of separation in a person's life, like puberty, junior year of high school (exploring going away from home), senior year (leaving home), freshman college year, marriage or childbirth. A despair over ever developing the dependency bond that would allow for accessibility to direct parental identity messages gives birth to a process that might be characterized by the following stages:

1. **Achievement:** Competing with other women for thinness to prove to one's self that one is strong enough to tolerate deprivation.
2. **Security System:** Being soothed and assured by rigid behavior patterns, including discomfort, that one is free of unmet interpersonal needs. Increasing rigidity and extending behavior patterns to combat anxiety.
3. **Secondary Gain:** Seeing others respond with increased attention and nurturance.
4. **Pseudofunctional Identity:** Perceiving one's symptoms as comprising identity and assertiveness.

By the time anorexia has become chronic, the person has reached the fourth stage and is difficult to treat. She does not experience herself as ill, but rather as having made for herself the least uncomfortable adjustment in what has become an emotionally painful existence.

Additionally, as the anorexic becomes more chronic, she becomes more preoccupied with issues of weight, eating, elimination, and appearance to the exclusion of more in-depth thoughts about self. There is practically no thinking about the future, either immediate or long-range, and little thought about interpersonal relationships, other than anger and guilt toward those she struggles with over her disease. Her needs deal only with the present, involving her bodily functions. Thoughts about relationships, with all their complexity, become a very low priority, pushed out of the conscious mind by obsessional constriction. Indeed, part of the rage experienced by family members toward the anorexic is not only related to her refusal to gain weight but toward her inability to relate to them and behave in an interpersonal manner. Members of the family often talk of their frustration, their desire to shake her by the shoulders and shout, "Is anybody there?" She is experienced as a vacant person, separated by her disfigured appearance and her glazed-over look. With chronic anorexia nervosa, family members often succumb to the victim's disengagement and withdraw from her in despair.

The cumulative effect of her mental self-neglect (and of the single-faceted relationship she and her family have evolved) deepens the sense of emptiness and insubstantiality. It is not surprising, then, that she would attempt to fill the disease-caused emptiness with a disease-fostered sense of identity-as-anorexic.

The frustrations expressed by the anorexic's family may also collectively fill the identity void that exists as a result of lack of direct parental identity messages. The anorexic, especially one who is chronic, hears all of her family's complaints about her disordered behavior as the most concrete way she has ever been recognized by them.

One patient who had recovered most of her weight became tearful when she was asked how she would feel about recovering her menstrual cycle. I inquired if the physical aspect of menstruating disturbed her.

She clarified, "No, I don't care about the physical part. It's the *meaning* of it."

"Are you afraid that you will be regarded as a woman? That more demands will be placed on you by others?"

She seemed surprised by my interpretation and corrected me. "No, no. I don't care about that. I just don't even think about it. But if my weight is normal and I get my period, then I'm not anorexic anymore. And that mean's I'm nothing, and everyone will forget about me."

What this young woman was saying is that *she* would have no way to view herself without the identity of the illness. It was a way of identifying herself that had been validated by those around her. A full recovery from anorexia nervosa must include the acquisition of a sense of identity to replace the sense of emptiness and the ability to tolerate the loss of the pseudo-functional identity. Anorexia nervosa is perhaps the most complex and seductive of the obsessional and obsessive-compulsive disorders.

One of the major controversies in the treatment of anorexia is the issue of addressing the symptoms directly. Positions taken on this issue range from a purely behavioristic approach, which addresses little more than the symptoms, to a general psycho-analytical approach in which the therapist refuses to address the symptoms at all in the belief that when the underlying conflicts are resolved, the symptoms will vanish. Both ends of the treatment spectrum exclude the patient's personality and the influence of the symptoms over that personality.

The case of Alice illustrates the employment of anorexia as a pseudofunctional identity by a young woman whose early development and physical-health problems made her vulnerable to just such a disorder. Alice was thirteen when she was fitted for a back brace for severe scoliosis. It was "a big boxlike affair," as she puts it. "It went from my shoulders to my hips. It made my body look like a rectangular cube. Ultimately it failed, and I needed spinal surgery."

Alice had vague recollections of her mother's many ailments, but since she was only eight when this began, she is unclear as to whether they were physical or psychological. She remembers an air of mystery about her mother's illness.

By Alice's early twenties, her mother had become mostly housebound. Alice's father died when she was nineteen. She was the last of four children, nine years younger than her brother, the third child. She felt that the family was tired by the time of her birth. Her father was involved with her medical problems but had little other focus on her. She remembered him as a sweet man who took a lot of trouble about her back.

Alice had severe asthma from five to twelve years of age, with numerous visits to the emergency room following hours of labored breathing. She remembers the oxygen and the Adrenalin injections and her parents standing over her bed, alarm on their faces.

Alice developed anorexia nervosa at fifteen. No one noticed for the first year. "Under the back brace, I could have looked like anything," Alice explains. "No one could tell." She sought treatment for her anorexia at the age of twenty-one. Prior to her seeking treatment, her family had expressed annoyance at her thinness and her peculiar eating habits. She ate low-calorie foods at measured intervals. She ate nothing until noon, when she had a light lunch, and then she had a light dinner at eight and a small snack before going to sleep.

Alice had never been hospitalized for anorexia nor received any professional attention for an eating problem. Her family grumbled about it but did not struggle with her, nor did they make a fuss when she picked at her fingertips until they bled or occasionally pulled out her hair, one strand at a time until her hair became thinner on the right side of her head. She also bit her lip, which showed chronic lacerations.

Alice had always done well in school and had been considered a tomboy before the back brace. She held a responsible job at the time she entered therapy, but she had no social activities except an occasional phone contact with a childhood friend. She was fully occupied with work and exercise. Her exercises were repetitious, rigid, ritualized. She could never do fewer than a specific number, only more. She was five feet six and weighted just ninety-one pounds. By the age of twenty-three, she had menstruated only twice in her life.

Despite the chronicity (six years) of her disorder, Alice was not defiant or defensive. She was curious about her condition and puzzled about herself and her strange behavior.

"I have to feel that I deserve to eat," she told me. "I won't eat unless I have been hungry for three or more hours. I have to swim for an hour every day. I never take the bus. I always walk unless I don't have the time to."

Although Alice was shy in therapy sessions, she could talk

about the facts of past events impersonally without difficulty. But when asked how she felt about a specific event in her life, for instance how she felt at the time something happened or in retrospect, she could not find words to answer. Even when asked how she was feeling at a particular moment during a therapy session, she would be perplexed by the question. She simply had no language with which to speak about her emotions. Although she was able to cry about issues that made her sad, she was not able to talk about that sadness.

It took two years of therapy before Alice could identify her feelings verbally and discuss them in the language this required. We had identified this problem in her first several sessions and agreed that teaching her to develop language about her feelings would be part of the therapy.

A major theme in Alice's treatment was that for her to release herself from her rituals and her rigid behavior patterns would create overwhelming anxiety and, sometimes, panic. After two years of therapy, Alice analyzed her anxiety this way: "When I was young, I was sick with asthma, then it was my back brace, then my surgery. I always knew who I was when I was sick, different from others, or in pain. The rest of the time, I felt invisible, not just to everyone else, but to me. I didn't know who I was when I wasn't identifiable by sickness, discomfort, or being unlike everyone else."

Alice experienced a great deal of awkwardness when she entered therapy. She said that it felt self-indulgent—almost greedy—for her to want the kind of personal attention that occurs in psychotherapy. She expressed her conflict about wanting the attention but feeling guilty about it: "It's easier being hungry," she said, "or in physical pain, or being fatigued than being here. It's almost more comfortable being uncomfortable . . . I don't know how to say it! It's just that I know who I am when I'm hungry or tired better than I know it here."

I asked her who she had been told she was while she was growing up. What words were used to identify her? What kind of comments were made about her? She seemed confused, and when she tried to answer, all she could come up with was, "selfish."

Alice felt guilty about saying even this. She explained that her parents were hardworking people; they had raised three children before she came along, and they had a right to an easier life. She had no recollection of conversations with her parents and could not remember ways in which they identified her personality or character traits. Her own sense of identity was derived from the way she related to her body and the kind of signals returned to her. If she starved, her stomach signaled her with hunger pains; if she swam hard, she felt fatigue. These signals told her that she was virtuous and not selfish.

Alice's system also included secrecy. When she first developed anorexia nervosa, she lived in a concealing back brace. She claims that her initial reason for losing weight was to prevent herself from outgrowing her back brace, which fit her like a body cast. Having been a tomboy in her elementary school years, she never coped with the development of her adolescent femininity. From puberty on, her body looked to the world like a rectangular cube. Since she could not display her emerging femininity, she adopted the role of the class clown. The back brace was the perfect costume. When the brace came off, Alice had a new special appearance to exhibit—an emaciated body.

Even while playing the clown, Alice had withdrawn her emotional connection to others. Her identity as she experienced it was nonsocial in origin. It was self-developed and obsessional in nature. Its continuance depended on relentless reenforcement of restrictive eating patterns, strenuous exercise, and low weight coupled with fatigue, cold, and pain as indicators of adequacy.

Alice is a good example of how self-destructive behavior becomes incorporated into a system of coping with one's sense of emptiness in an obsessive-compulsive syndrome such as anorexia nervosa. Thinking about the trials of Alice's adolescent development and the lonely isolation she experienced, it is possible to understand how great a discrepancy can exist between the obsessive person's conviction that her behaviors are essential to her existence and the recognition of their self-destructiveness. To Alice, and others like her, these dangerous routines and rituals—this adherence to rigidity and perfection—are all she has to provide her with a sense of identity.

After five years of treatment, Alice diminished her dependence on rituals by 80 percent but her OCD took a large chunk out of her young adulthood.

BULIMIA NERVOSA

While the anorexic's behaviors are conceived as her identity, the bulimic's behavior serves more of a secret regulatory function. Binging and vomiting, as well as laxative abuse, become the hidden regulators of anxiety, panic, and depression. While the anorexic openly presents family and friends with a new personality (the disfigured appearance, the willpower to deprive herself, the extensive eating rituals), the bulimic hides her rituals and attempts to pretend nothing at all has changed. An examination of bulimia can help us understand this area of secrecy—of hidden rituals—as it applies to the wider spectrum of obsessional behavior.

Bulimia nervosa is defined* as:

1. Recurrent episodes of binge eating (rapid consumption of a large amount of food in a short period of time).
2. A feeling of lack of control over eating behavior during the eating binges.
3. Engaging regularly in either self-induced vomiting, the use of laxatives or diuretics, strict dieting or fasting, or vigorous exercise in order to prevent weight gain.

*Diagnostic and Statistical Manual of Mental Disorders, 3rd ed. (American Psychiatric Association).

4. A minimum average of two binge-eating episodes per week for at least three months.

5. Persistent overconcern with body weight and shape.

Considering the behaviors listed above, it is natural to have questions as to their cause. Most bulimics are themselves puzzled about their excessive drive to eat, except to note that it intensifies when they are upset. Many bulimics engage in multisubstance abuse; that is, they also may abuse alcohol, narcotics, sedatives, sleeping pills, diet pills, and laxatives. Despite their daily periods of emotional chaos, bulimics are often highly organized, successful women who expend prodigious amounts of energy in jobs and careers. Their food abuse is usually contained and confined to a time of day when they have the privacy required for this addictive behavior toward food.

If obsessionality is boundless overthinking about security-making ideas and behaviors, then the bulimic's food addiction may be seen as contained obsessionality. It is contained in the sense that it is self-limited because of a greater sense of personality and identity (certainly greater than anorexics), which limits the need for self-soothing behaviors. While there may be some difficulty with a cohesive sense of sexual identity, this is usually more developed than in the anorexic. And although bulimics suffer from a sense of separateness and emptiness similar to that of anorexics, this usually develops in bulimics at a later age.

The bulimic forms rigid behavior patterns with regard to eating, purging, and elimination, but these are confined to specific parts of her day, which allows her to live a normal-appearing existence; however, the time and secrecy necessary for this binging and purging causes the bulimic to be subtly disconnected from her family and friends. Ashamed of her secret obsession with food, she must posture in an outgoing and overly pleasing manner so that her disconnection is barely detectable by those around her.

In comparing bulimia with anorexia, it should be noted that

both create emotional withdrawal, rigidity, obsessional thinking, and, eventually, a sense of eroding identity. But those who
develop bulimia come from a broader spectrum of personality
types and extended variation in degree of disorder than do
those who develop anorexia. Actually, those bulimics who most
closely resemble stereotypical victims of anorexia are those who
evolved bulimic patterns from anorexia nervosa. If the reverse
occurs—if one is bulimic and then becomes anorexic, so that
body image becomes a mainstay of the ritualistic system—it is
probable that the pseudofunctional identity of the anorexic will
become a threat to the more developed identity system that the
bulimic may have achieved.

How does the bulimic's pattern of behavior begin? Why
would any obsessional personality in search of reassurance
(rituals) choose such grotesque conduct as binging and purging, gorging and vomiting? The answer sometimes is that the
potential bulimic has a potential addiction to food (the purge,
then, acting only as an enabling factor) in the same way one
may have a potential addiction to alcohol. If this is the case, the
bulimic's special pattern addiction may be a bridge between
traditional substance abusers and those with obsessive-
compulsive disorders. Pattern addiction is the irresistible compulsion to repeat behaviors with substances that have no
identifiably addictive properties. In somewhat the same way
that many alcoholics have started drinking casually in social
settings, bulimics may embark on their obsessive conduct with
no sense of its potential addictiveness. Consider the case of
Veronica and the vomiting trick.

When we met, Veronica was thirty years of age. All her teeth
had been capped, and some had needed a second capping due
to continued gum recession and exposed enamel, ripe for
decay, a result of hydrochloric acid eroding away the tooth
enamel.

"I had vomited for twelve years, until two years ago," she told
me. "It all started in boarding school, in dance class. We would
all go out for pizza, stuffing ourselves. We knew that the dance
teacher would be displeased if we gained weight. In dance, you

have to be thin enough for the men to carry you without looking awkward. You had to be a graceful dancer and double as lightweight baggage. I had been putting on a few pounds, not proper in a British boarding school. Well, one night I protested the pizza feast. The girls looked at me conspiratorially, and Cynthia started giggling. She told me, 'You don't have to gain weight, silly. There's the *trick*.'

"I was puzzled. 'What trick?' I asked.

"They looked at each other and resumed giggling. In a chorus, they all opened their mouths wide and pointed with their index fingers. I still didn't understand. Were they pointing to their teeth, their tonsils? In unison, they replied, 'Vomiting.'

"They called it gang vomiting. Sometimes we did it within sight of each other, sometimes in parallel stalls in the ladies' room, and sometimes we just stood in a line, waiting for that one, overworked toilet. We might draw lots before we ate to see who would go first through eighth, knowing that the last to throw up would gain the most weight from what she ate. At least we thought so.

"Well, it all seemed so social, so peer-group oriented, as they say here in the States. We didn't realize until years after graduation that five of the eight of us were still gang vomiting without the gang—stuck in this pattern, ruining our teeth, and feeling crazy with this thing that came to be called bulimia. We didn't know it could become a disease, but it certainly did for us.

"We simply couldn't stop. I think we were ashamed to admit it to ourselves, much like problem drinkers, I suppose. We didn't seem so much alike when it all started. I mean, we came from different sorts of families. We had different temperaments, different degrees of sociability. Diana was a positive introvert. Claire was always outgoing—partying, I think the kids call it today. Eunice was serious, but could be outgoing or solitary. Well, anyway, all we had in common was the dance class . . . and the trick."

Without more information about the personality and background of each of these women, it is not possible to explain why some had the strength to relinquish the pattern of binging and purging while the others remained trapped within it. However, it is known that binge-purge behavior utilized chronically will become part of anxiety-depression regulation and be incorporated into a defense mechanism as are other obsessive-compulsive rituals. It will, in most cases, erode an individual's ability to maintain intimacy, and gradually create and increase the sense of emptiness described in the character development of most sufferers of obsessive-compulsive disorders.

Researchers have demonstrated the effectiveness of the use of certain antidepressants in stopping binge-purge behavior, which suggests that unrecognized depression is one factor in predisposing some toward this behavior. Many bulimics report a feeling of panic before they begin to eat, and the behavior of binging followed by purging appears to block the panic and anxiety as well as depression and feelings of emptiness. One researcher, Dr. Hans Huebner, suggests that the body's sudden discharge of gastric fluids (due to binging) triggers the release of endorphins, the body's natural pain killers, which create a sense of temporary well-being and that the binge-purge sequence, in effect, makes the individual high.*

With both anorexia nervosa and bulimia, certain deficits in identity development may be present at the illness's onset. Depression, anxiety, and panic disorder may be present as well, either as constitutional factors (a hereditary predisposition which is biochemical in nature), or as psychodynamic, the effects of a family system on the individual. From the standpoint of this study, what is of special importance is the fact that any obsessional personality who engages in a pattern of anorexia or bulimia faces a very high probability of fully developing the disease. And this will lead inevitably to a worsening of the individual's condition, for feelings of emptiness, tendencies toward obsessionality, rigidity, and emotional withdrawal from

*Lecture, Albert Einstein International Conference on Eating Disorders, New York, 1986.

others all will be intensified by the disordered eating patterns and their accompanying biological malnutrition and erratic nutrition.

Eating disorders greatly increase the complexity of recovery for a person with an obsessive-compulsive disorder. The eating disorder becomes the most intense cluster of obsessional behaviors and has to be treated first, since other defenses are less dangerous. Eating disorders can become permanent—and even fatal.

SIX

The Cleanliness
Defense

Although the repetitive behavior of OCD takes many forms, including exercise, checking locks, counting, folding clothes, and rearranging furniture, perhaps the oldest form known to the public as well as mental health professionals is handwashing. It is also one of the most enlightening for a general understanding of OCD because of the relative obviousness of cause and effect.

One might speculate that this particular disorder became more prolific during the nineteenth century when scientists discovered that the cause of disease, as opposed to bodily breakdown or malfunction, which suggested a "mechanical failure," was actually microorganisms that somehow entered the body. People who were anxious were provided with a perfect target for their anxieties—germs—and it was a target that came with a convenient behavioral solution: repetitive handwashing.

When I was first studying psychology in 1960, obsessive-compulsive disorders were considered incurable but also of very little consequence. If someone was a compulsive hand-washer, so the thinking went, just give them some hand cream.

But then along came anorexia nervosa, which certainly looks and sounds like one form of obsessive-compulsive disorder, and health specialists could not simply give OCDs hand cream anymore. People were starving to death. They had to have tubes put in their noses and chests and all sorts of other extreme measures to keep them alive. So suddenly it became important to understand the underlying causes of obsessive-compulsive disorders, including those with a cleanliness defense.

The compulsive handwasher is continually concerned with contamination. Most, but not all, of this behavior is centered around the bathroom and eating. In the bathroom, one is concerned with both contamination from others (who have been there previously) and from one's own body (urinary tract and anus). In addition to being contaminated by urine or fecal material, one worries about both orifices being the entry point for invading contaminants. Normal personal hygiene requires that one keep these areas free of exretory residue and avoid exposure to unclean conditions. The sufferer of a compulsive cleanliness disorder carries personal hygiene far beyond appropriateness.

We have already discussed Linda and the extensive amount of time she was forced to devote to her bathroom routine. But the obsession with cleanliness often leads to problems outside the bathroom as well as within. Consider Paul, a thirty-year-old computer designer who lived with his parents and younger brother. Paul was a quiet child who always did exceptionally well in school but not well in sports.

Although it is not possible to pinpoint the onset of his OCD behavior, it is known that beginning with the fourth grade (age nine), Paul refused to leave the classroom to play ball in the backyard. Instead, he remained inside, fearing that the backyard was dirty, and his teacher noticed that he washed his hands a half dozen times during the one-hour recess period. His parents were notified about this, but they requested that the school overlook his behavior. The school complied with their wishes and excused Paul from outdoor activity.

For Paul's tenth birthday, he requested his own vacuum cleaner. His parents thought that this was an unusual request, but it did not seem dangerous and offered some real benefit, since the family did not have any help with housecleaning. Paul cleaned his room several times a day with his gift. At some point, his parents noticed that he began to wash the walls of his room. When questioned about this, Paul claimed that the walls had grease on them.

Within a year, Paul rarely ventured out of his room while at home. He only entered the kitchen when no one else was there. He no longer used utensils to eat his food; rather, he handled the food with plastic wrap. His parents were distressed at this and bought him plastic throwaway gloves to eat with. The family "always regarded Paul as a tense child," his mother said, "and we just didn't want to make things worse by fighting him on these habits."

Paul's mother described herself as a nervous person who prefered to spend most of her time at home. She was actually an agoraphobic who became anxious the moment she left her house and was terrified at the prospect of riding in a car. It is not surprising that she provided no strong parental support for Paul's early years or that she was unable to confront him when his cleanliness obsession became obvious.

Of her husband, she said, "He's a kind man, but he can't stand up to people. He's always been taken advantage of in business." As a parent, Paul's father was detached and timid, never confrontational, never able to provide the authoritative role so desperately needed by Paul.

Together, the mother and father made up what is termed a conflict-avoidance family. Although they were physically present to offer support in some form, there was no substantiality. Holding his parents' nurturing in low esteem, Paul turned inward for reassurance and to ritualized repetition based on cleanliness.

Over the years, Paul's fear of contamination deepened. He bought his own mini washer and dryer at the age of thirteen, and became virtually a hermit. By the time he sought treatment for his disorder, he had been limited by it for twenty-one years. His adult life was restricted to going to work, cleaning his clothes, and washing the walls of his room. He had covered the walls with white paint so he could see any dirt that might accumulate, and he had to use glossy enamel because he literally washed off any other paint down to the plaster. His foods were all frozen in plastic wrappers that were boiled, and he used large numbers of plastic throwaway gloves each day. Although he relinquished his rituals when he went to work, he always showered for long periods of time as soon as he returned home.

Paul was aware that his parents were increasingly absent from his emotional life as he drifted deeper and deeper into his expanded obsessive-compulsive repertoire of ideas and behaviors. But when asked how he felt about these behaviors and how much he wanted to be rid of them, he responded with ambivalence: "I can't stand how much of my life is dominated by the rituals," he acknowledged, "but at the same time, I don't know what I would do if they were gone. I mean, I would be mentally and emotionally empty without them. There's just work. There are no people in my life. I haven't felt close to my family since I was a little kid, if ever. I don't like my life, but I don't know what to exchange it for."

Despite the ambivalence, Paul finally did, of his own volition, seek help for his obsessive-compulsive behaviors. What prompted this change? Why, after so many years bound by rituals and emotional isolation, did he finally make a move to be rid of them? The change came about as a result of a combination of factors. Concerned with numbers, Paul's thirtieth birthday meant to him that he might never have a normal life, and this made him more desperate. There was also the fact that his father had suffered a heart attack and was deteriorating, and at that point the whole issue of how much Paul's parents could continue to support his OCD—indeed, how long his parents would live and his world remain unchanged—began to frighten Paul, making him extremely anxious and even, at times, panicky.

It was this constant state of anxiety and panic plus increasing depression about the chronicity of his OCD and his despair about ever overcoming it that finally brought Paul to therapy.

During our first session, I noticed that as he walked into the room, he seemed to notice more than most people. As a matter of fact, he was so observant that he fixed his eyes on the carpeting, curtains, furniture, and paintings. Only then, after taking in every detail of the room, did he sit down. This whole process took him several very conspicuous minutes.

When he was seated, I asked Paul if he was always so observant about environments that he entered.

He looked at me and then answered slowly, "It's not just a matter of being observant. I have to do a lot of thinking about every place I enter."

"What kind of thinking did you have to do as you entered this room?"

He was hesitant. But after keeping all those secrets for so many years, he was determined to tell his story, no matter what the inner cost. He looked at me, glanced down at the carpet, then looked back and said, finally, "I'm very busy mentally when I come into a new room like your office. I have to look at everything carefully. I not only have to *look* at everything— every piece of furniture and where the doors and windows are located—but I have to think about them all, imagine them in my mind. If I don't do that, I feel something terrible will happen. It's simply unthinkable to not do that."

"Doesn't that make your life difficult?" I asked. "It must slow you down quite a bit."

He nodded. "Oh, yes, especially at work, if I have to go to a new office or company. That's one of the reasons I hate to change jobs."

"Do other people notice the way you look at things?"

"Yes. They wonder why I stare. But even though I know they'll wonder, I don't have any choice. I have to take in every new place I go into."

I asked, "Did you have to take in every detail of my appearance as well as objects in the room?"

He laughed quietly and responded, "Not really. People don't count in my pictures. It's only the other objects I have to think about. Actually, it may take me months to remember what you look like."

Paul spent the first four months of his therapy cataloguing his obsessive-compulsive disorders, the history of them and when they developed. It was after the fourth month that I asked him to begin to focus on how he felt talking to me in this office and what that meant to him.

He found himself unable to answer, and was taken aback. He had been so informative about his OCD rituals. He had been able to tell me when they developed and how one led to another and how many times he performed each one. So now he was distressed at his inability to respond when I asked how he felt in talking about all this with another person, in other words, how he felt about me.

After a long pause, he said, "I really try hard not to notice you as much as possible." He did not appear embarrassed at what seemed a rejection of me. "But I'm that way with every-one. I try to not be aware of people. I have a great deal of difficulty talking about my feelings toward people. In fact I have a hard time talking about my feelings about anything. It's not that I don't want to. I mean, I came here to get help, to talk to you. And if feels okay to do that. But I don't know how to talk about my feelings in being here or how I feel about talking to you."

He missed his next session, having called and said work was keeping him too busy, but the real reason was probably his desire to postpone any discussion about his feelings concerning himself, his family, and his therapy. Nevertheless, he soon returned to treatment, finally managing to talk about his feelings after I was able to supply him with a new language. (This element of treatment will be explained in chapter 9, "Talking.")

Later I asked Paul about his involvement with women. He said, "I try not to have any real contact with them, not to care about them. I'm sure being interested in them will only get me in trouble."

"Why?"

"Well, women know that we're attracted to them. They know that we want to be sexually involved with them, and they can take advantage of our need to be sexually attached. They can take advantage and use that to control us, and I can't stand being controlled by anyone. So I have an interest in women, but I keep it to myself. I don't have anything to do with women."

I asked Paul if these feelings made him angry at women.

"No," he said. "They don't make me angry. I don't believe women think about me. I don't believe they're out to get me. I just feel that women would make me too vulnerable, and I'm not prepared to be close to anyone or even to take the chance of being controlled by anyone. And women would be able to do that to me. So I just simply stay away from them."

After almost four years of treatment, psychotherapy and medication, that situation changed dramatically. Paul had a dating relationship (bordering on a live-in relationship) with a woman his own age. He was also virtually free of all his rituals.

SEVEN
False Assumptions

What is the therapist's role in psychotherapy? The typical portrayal on television or in the movies has the therapist limited to sitting in a chair beside the couch, listening a bit distractedly to the patient's stream of consciousness; and if the patient should ask, "What does it mean when I do that?" the therapist responds, "What do *you* think it means?"

If this portrayal was ever accurate, it is no longer. The accumulation of evidence demonstrating the success of more active participation by the therapist has demanded change. A friend of mine, a psychoanalytically trained psychiatrist practicing for twenty years, recently remarked to me about her treatment of a middle-aged agoraphobic patient: "She was losing weight because she was afraid to leave her home to go shopping, so I decided to take her food shopping as part of her therapy. I enjoyed taking care of her. It made me feel good, and I used her therapeutic connection to me as a way of desensitizing her to her fear of going out. We spent a lot of time analyzing how it felt for her to go shopping with me. I also knew that she had had enough to eat when she came to her next therapy session, so I wasn't anxious about doing the necessary confrontation about her eating at certain points in the session. It's something I couldn't have done ten years ago, but I trust myself as an analyst enough to do whatever I believe is right for my patients."

My friend's phrase, "taking care of her," is not a phrase that sits well with many psychotherapists. Perhaps it suggests an inappropriately parental posture, or something seductive, or dominating. And many therapists, especially those who have not been practicing for a long time, have concerns about creating emotional involvement and dependency on the part of patients.

Although the phrase "taking care of patients" is familiar to a medical school graduate, the concepts of physical care and psychological care seem to have little in common. Society recognizes that physicians have a responsibility for the physical well-being of a patient as a result of what they have or have not done medically. It is a legal and financial liability as well. No such recognition has been made yet for the therapist and the mental well-being of patients. Perhaps as a result of the plethora of malpractice suits, some psychotherapists are becoming more conservative and will shun any explicit responsibility for caretaking other than as facilitating listeners. After all, who wants to get sued for giving bad advice? But as simply a facilitating listener, the therapist is not likely to help at least one group of patients: those suffering from obsessive-compulsive disorders. Why? Because success for the facilitating listener demands good candidates for psychotherapy, and OCDs do not fit that category.

Consider the assumptions made about individuals who are seen as good candidates for psychotherapy. One belief is that they are willing to engage in a relationship where they are the recipient of help. A second is that they need the autonomy to compensate (they have to feel responsible for the success of the therapy), perhaps for the oppression by others in their lives, or at least for the oppression by the ideas of others in their thoughts and feelings. A third assumption is that the person seeking treatment—the person who enters therapy with complaints about his or her emotional makeup—has a collection of ideas to present.

The obsessional patient often brings none of these to therapy—no willingness to be the recipient of help, no need to compensate for oppressive parents, not even a fund of ideas about self. This makes the normal patient-therapist relationship almost impossible if meaningful progress is to be made, as an examination of each of these assumptions makes quite clear.

1. The first assumption about individuals who are good candidates for psychotherapy is that as patients they should be willing to engage in a relationship where they are the recipient of help.

This is such an obvious requisite that initiating psychotherapy without it seems virtually impossible. Yet the obsessive-compulsive patient is not ready or willing to engage. True, these patients come to therapy ostensibly seeking help, but very often a major part of their need is to overcome inaccessibility! Their symptoms have communicated a need to be helped, but the patients have no language with which to speak about how these symptoms came into being. And even if they could find the words to explain their situation, far from being overtly dependent personalities, ready to lay their burdens upon another, they consider any sort of dependency to be unvirtuous, dangerous, and competitive with the security offered by their rituals—the obsessional defenses that require emotional isolation to work. Indeed, the moment even the slightest dependency is employed, it becomes hostile dependency, for it makes the patients feel helpless and emotionally shut off from the service of their obsessive-compulsive defenses.

Obsessional patients do come to therapy with what is known as the forbidden wish to be the recipient of help. But this is the wish they first denied in early childhood and have continued to deny ever since. Patient defenses against this forbidden wish include the mistrust they feel for others, which leads to fears of being abandoned by any helper, including the therapist. "If I'm going to be abandoned," the patient reasons, "why should I even hope to trust?" Thus the therapist is an unwanted partner, a necessary evil barely tolerated by the patient in order to eliminate behaviors and thoughts that have become almost overpowering.

Rather than meeting individuals willing to engage in a relationship, the therapist who first encounters OCDs finds seemingly unreachable or hostile patients who abhor any display of dependency in themselves. There is no reaching out on the part of the patients. All the therapist can hope to build upon is that forbidden wish that has the patients implicitly delivering the rather forlorn and paradoxical message, "Help me to stop stopping you from helping me."

2. A second assumption about individuals who are good candidates for psychotherapy is that they need autonomy to compensate, perhaps for the oppression by others in their lives.

This assumption makes the patient a good candidate because it indicates the patient's need for controlling the therapy sessions; for opening up, a desire on the patient's part to get out from under an oppressive thumb and express his or her thoughts and feelings to someone who shows interest and appreciation. But there has been no such oppression for OCDs. On the contrary, I have found that most patients suffering from obsessional disorders are characterized as under-parented. Rather than offering descriptions of tyrannical parents, they are apt to tell the therapist that their parents were exhausted or depleted. The style of parent-child interaction was either passive-dependent or intrusive-dependent. In either case, the child never lost sight of the parents as used-up and deferential to the child, clearly the opposite of oppressive. There is, then, no thumb from which to escape and no hunger for autonomy and self-expression.

If the patient's parents were intrusive-dependent, the therapist faces a second pitfall. If he follows the usual procedure in psychotherapy, asking background questions during the initial interview, he may be replaying, in the patient's eyes, the dependent parent. Often inquiring and displaying a need to be part of everything the child does or thinks, such parents seem to be assigning to the patient responsibility for the family's well-being, as in the cliché, "You're destroying this family." If the therapist begins treatment with intrusive questions, he may be seen as assigning the patient personal responsibility for the success or failure of the therapy—this to a patient who is already overly responsible!

3. A third assumption about individuals who are good candidates for psychotherapy is that the person who enters treatment with complaints about his or her emotional makeup has a collection of ideas to present.

As stated earlier, perhaps the chief characteristic of obsessional patients is a sense of emptiness due largely to an insufficiency of parental identity messages and often characterized by statements such as, "I feel like nobody . . . I am nothing . . . I feel like there's nobody inside . . . I just try to be like whoever I'm with at the time." It is totally unrealistic to expect such empty individuals to bring with them to therapy a collection of ideas to present.

If the therapist chooses to probe for such ideas at the outset, he may immediately increase the patient's resistance to therapy. Obsessional patients will interpret the therapist's questions as indicative of neediness. "Help me to understand you," might be what obsessional ears hear in the therapist's questions, and obsessional patients are contemptuous of those who need help, especially if they are officially designated caretakers (parents, teachers, supervisors). If more open-ended questions requiring long answers are asked, patients may feel, along with contempt, a sense of abandonment as they are left alone on the stage to perform for the therapist.

None of these feelings will be expressed by the new patients, who may despairingly accept the role of informing (taking care of) the therapist. Viewing the therapist as needy within their own mistrustful framework, the patients now view themselves as both nurturing and authoritative. This provokes their transferential response of despair and contempt. Often such patients will attend several sessions, produce lots of material, and then disappear after providing a diplomatic reason for termination (to protect the needy therapist).

EIGHT

The Therapist's Role

Because those suffering from obsessive-compulsive disorders are not good candidates for psychoanalytical psychotherapy, they demand far more active participation on the part of the therapist. What should he or she do?

1. Take the initiative.

The first phase of treatment is the most interpersonal, and the least distant for the therapist. It is here that he must take the initiative to help the patient enter into an alliance. The therapist might begin with a simple explanation.

Many people entering treatment do not know how therapy works and may be too embarrassed to ask. It is fair and helpful to explain how one person in the room is going to help the other. It is not uncommon for the therapist to inform the patient, "Your obligations here are to keep your appointments and to pay your bills." Fair enough; but what about stating what the therapist's obligations are to the patient? In the past, these have been unstated, allowed to remain implicit, acquire mystery, create a blank slate for the patient to project upon. For the patient entering therapy with feelings of emptiness, mistrust, and obsessional defenses, such an analytic posture will simply drive the patient deeper into self-soothing defenses and create additional resistance to treatment.

Instead, why not begin by establishing who is responsible for the conduct of the therapy? And what about its outcome? Might the therapist not at least state that he will try to help the patient? Guarantees would be grandiose, but a declaration of earnest intention to help the troubled person overcome problems seems reasonable enough. And rather than the traditional, "You are the kind of person who can benefit from psychotherapy," I suggest, "I think I may be able to help you with your problem." This lets the patient know that a fair share of the responsibility has been placed upon the therapist. The former statement seems self-serving in that the therapist or analyst explicitly opts for very little responsibility for the outcome. To the patient who is obsessional and empty, the blank slate of an analytic therapist might be just one more insubstantial adult too passive to offer help.

In the case of twenty-three-year-old Ashley, whom we met earlier and who exhibited excessive exercise compulsions, I clearly needed to take the initiative. In our initial session, she indicated to me, "I have all this compulsive behavior I have to get rid of." She was letting me know that her symptom needed to be treated, but she was not at all sure that she could envision herself as the recipient of care in a psychotherapeutic relationship, or any relationship for that matter. Generally, she began each session by saying, "I'm okay today." She would then enumerate all the positives that had occurred in the few days prior to the session and conclude her opening comments with, "Well, what do you want to talk about today?"

Her behavior was an attempt to reverse roles with me. She presented herself as needing no help and asking me what my needs were for the session. It is important to examine what is happening in such sessions in order to reduce this resistance, which rather deftly maneuvers to make the therapist feel unnecessary and inadequate.

"Why are you asking me what I'd like to talk about today?"

"I want you to ask me more specific questions," she said. "I can answer those better."

"All right. Have you spoken with your parents on the phone?"

"Yes. They're the usual. Just complaining about each other."

"How does that affect you?"

"You know how Daddy can reduce me to tears, but there's nothing I can do about it. That's part of the usual, too." This was followed by nervous laughter.

"Why are you laughing?" I asked her.

"You know . . . It's my cover-up. I don't want to cry, so I laugh." She shrugged her shoulders and continued to smile.

"What do you think is happening here right now?"

"What do you mean?"

"You have reassured me that you're fine," I told her. "You laugh nervously and interpret your laughter for me. I might think you're trying to tell me that there's very little I have to offer you, and yet I believe you came here in the hope that I can break through all your protests."

"Well, of course I do." She shrugged her shoulders and looked scolded for a moment. Her pace then picked up. "You know how dangerous it is for me to trust anyone. If I take a chance, which I do repeatedly with my father, he verbally rips me to shreds until I'm completely reduced to tears. So how can you ask me to do that with you?"

"Well, that's better. It's better that you have dropped your self-mocking tone."

"Do I get a gold star?" She responded sarcastically, with accompanying laughter.

"Ah," I said. "So it's too painful to remain accessible for more than a brief moment."

"You know that it is . . . for me."

I nodded. "Then we will make it our priority to lengthen the time span of your vulnerability here."

"But you know how hard that is for me."

"Yes. So we'll both work very hard on it."

Clearly, we were discussing our relationship within therapy. We had gone beyond what might be termed an analysis of the transference; the tone of the session was highly interpersonal. An analytical dialogue would have eliminated the therapist's use of "I, me, and we."

I employ self-referential pronouns whenever possible (and reasonable) to emphasize that psychotherapy is an interpersonal process. For individuals who have difficulty engaging in any sort of relationship, intimacy, or attachment, and whose pathology may originate with that difficulty (or failure), this approach is simultaneously uncomfortable and attracting.

Obsessional personalities always resent the separateness that their self-reassuring system perpetuates. They look down upon all individuals they regard as weaker than themselves. On some level, that resentment can be traced back to child-parent relationships. In Ashley's case, she clung to the parents who she claims she has managed since she was a child. If she relinquished her role as their nurturer, then she had no identity. Her level of anxiety became significantly increased if she could not nurture within an important relationship. Yet she wanted help to relinquish this demanding function in its intensely compelling form. She understood that if she could release herself from that role, she would be able to utilize the support of others, something that she had not been able to do in the past. It is the responsibility of the therapist to take the initiative and bring this out into the open, defining the roles for the two people involved.

Many therapists have expressed their own anxiety with regard to analyzing the here and now, or what I like to call "What's happening between the two people in the room." This is because the issues of interpersonal analysis, and the explicit assuming of responsibility for the direction of the psychotherapy, are usually left up to the patient. Therapists feel guilty if they believe they are being too directive with a patient. The result for many therapists is that when they intuitively feel that it might be in the patient's best interest to guide them, they do so guiltily, unconsciously, and therefore without sufficient planning. The patient experiences that therapist's guilt, perceives the therapist's vulnerability, and feels that he or she (the patient) is being too much of a burden to the therapist. This reinforces the patient's characteristic fear that dependency is unvirtuous and can harm the caretaker (the therapist, in this case).

Therefore the therapist must not only take the initiative, he must hold on to it.

2. Structure a nurturant-authoritative relationship.

Explicitly stating the therapist's responsibility for the treatment and making a declaration of intent—"I think I may be able to help you with your problem" or, later on, "We will make it our priority to lengthen the time span of your vulnerability here"—is implicitly providing nurturance within the therapeutic relationship as well as establishing an authoritative role. Typically, parents of the patient have not been experienced as authoritative. By the therapist's authoritative structuring, he or she preempts the patient's transferential expectations and disarms the patient's deflecting mechanism and resistance. Deprived of the ability to deflect, the patient may begin experiencing the forbidden wish for dependency and trust. This wish has been repressed since childhood for a variety of dynamic reasons within the family system. If, in experiencing this wish, the patient now becomes engaged in treatment and risks trust and dependency, the attachment can be used therapeutically to compensate the patient for the failure of childhood trust that led to the development of obsessional defenses. The attachment will also provide a deepening of transference on the part of the patient.

If this psychotherapy is termed reparenting, it may not sound professional enough, so, instead, it can be identified by the behaviors that compensate for the patient's heretofore unmet needs: nurturant-authoritative psychotherapy. The initial phase of this treatment is fraught with anxiety for obsessional patients because they are placed in conflict. Feeling at ease in the nurturing role themselves, they can also be effective at dominating a conversation. Now, as the therapist begins establishing a nurturant-authoritative role, the patients do not know who to be to the therapist. Since most obsessional individuals only experience trust as forbidden wish, there is severe ambivalence toward the therapist who is tempting them. But this ambivalence is valuable in treatment since it mobilizes the patient to become emotionally involved with the therapist, thus breaking out of the closed safe obsessional system.

Diane, a young woman in her twenties who had been in an automobile accident that partially disfigured her, had become obsessive-compulsive and found that her entire day was ritualized. She had become a weight-lifter, and she swaggered into my office for our first meeting. Sitting down, she placed her right hand across her face with her index finger crossing under her nose, with one raised eyebrow in a highly judgmental posture.

I looked at this display of bravado and responded with one raised eyebrow, nodding my head. "When I think of all the time and energy you are going to require—years of it—I could get tired just at the thought."

She looked surprised, dropped the swagger posture, raised both her eyebrows in astonishment, and responded in a loud, high-pitched protest, "You're scaring the shit out of me!"

"Then I guess you're planning to stick around for it."

She was relieved that she had lost the contest for dominance. She also understood that I perceived the forbidden wish that her entire posture denied. Implicitly interpreting patients' behavior, then, is part of the therapeutic repertoire necessary to cope with obsessional resistances. Explicit interpretation at this juncture would have given a message of dependence.

If I had responded to Diane's swaggering gait with, "You appear highly confident," or, "Your gait seems pronounced and dominant," I would have had a poor result. These observations, although noncritical, would have been heard by Diane as the therapist still needing verification from the patient. She had been testing me to see if I would be one more adult who would fail her by deferring to her and behaving dependently and therefore leaving her to feel abandoned.

If my interventions imply that I need the patient's help, then the patient will see me as one more dependent, abandoning parent. The transferential expectations that obsessional patients present (expectations that reinforce their resistance) are contempt for the weaker parent; fears that if one finds out how empty they are, one will lose interest in them; fears that if they lose control of their stability, no one will be able to retrieve them from emotional chaos. In other words, they fear that their caretakers lack both strength to employ on their behalf and empathy to their sense of inadequacy.

Throughout the early phase of treatment, it is vitally important for the therapist to keep much of the therapeutic process—the here and now—explained and interpreted, especially the patient's ambivalence. If the patient's threshold of anxiety should be overwhelmed by the therapeutic process, the patient will either feel chaotic or lost, or leave treatment, or both.

3. Build a bridge.

Many obsessional patients enter therapy complaining about themselves. "I hate myself," is a common complaint. This is usually misleading to the therapist. The temptation is to ask, "What is so terrible about you?" But when the patient states, "I hate myself," it is actually a complaint about her mental processes. What she means is, "I hate the way my mind works," or, "I hate the way I think," or, "I hate how badly I feel most of the time." While the complaint often sounds like a social or moral self-condemnation, it is, in fact, a complaint about the patient's characteristic mental postures and states of feeling.

Another frequent complaint heard in the beginning stages of therapy is one already mentioned: "I am nothing." Sometimes this may refer to lack of advancement in early adult tasks (for example, a young woman who has not married or found a suitable job or career). More often, however, the patient is complaining that she experiences emptiness; an inadequate sense of identity, an absence of a sense of self, an inability to develop a sense of purpose or direction.

Both of the complaints, "I hate myself" and "I am nothing," often represent a state of detachment, inertia, and confusion. The detachment is interpersonal and is a result of the patient's inaccessibility. It all but eliminates interpersonal dialogues and any motivation to focus on personal growth. If the detachment is severe enough, a chronic, internal, circular dialogue develops about most situations in a person's life that self-deceives the person on all issues and resolves none. The resulting chronic inertia fosters confusion, depression, and, often, reclusive behavior.

Since all this is an outcome of detachment, it is the therapist's task to bridge it. If this detachment is a reaction to the patient's viewing his or her parents as insubstantial, unnurturing, and contemptible, then the therapist's first job is to make certain he is not viewed in the same way. And he can only do this by displaying conduct that thwarts the patient's expectation that the therapist will be like the patient's parents.

As an example, let us return to the patient's complaint, "I am nothing." Rather than responding, "No, you're not," or asking the patient, "What do you think that means?" the therapist must take an active role, perhaps responding with, "If it is true that you're nothing now, then we'll have to develop within you a feeling of identity."

The emphasis in this kind of response is more on the therapist than the patient. It offers something concrete the therapist should be able to accomplish in place of just hope or hyperbole. The patient, however, will not be convinced by a new therapist who is overly optimistic about the patient's future. The only valid optimism the new therapist can present is self-confidence about his or her ability to help the patient. Properly presented, this can be enough to bridge the detachment.

4. Accept patient dependency.

The successful emergence of a sense of identity and the ability to form intimate relationships develop from a successful period of dependency during childhood. A failure in the period of early dependency results in the mistrust of others, a lack of sense of one's self (identity), and, eventually, the development of obsessional rituals. Since the disorders evolve from an early failure of dependency, the therapist's task is to compensate the individual with a successful period of therapeutic dependency.

Many therapists find it difficult to offer such compensation. The words to express allowance for the patient's utilization of dependency are missing in the vocabulary of many therapists, especially those who have not been practicing for a long time. This results in therapists' fears about their rescue impulses toward a particular patient, and they tend to analyze what it was in the patient's neurosis that provoked the rescue impulse. Far more benefit would accrue to the patient if the therapist would analyze instead how much dependency might be tactically and advisably offered to the patient. When a therapist experiences the impulse to rescue a patient and represses it, what usually happens is that the therapist compensates by overidentifying with the patient and temporarily abandoning his separate helping role, thereby fostering still more fear of dependency in the patient.

On the other hand, if the therapist has previously thought through his rescue role and is ready to accept predetermined limits on dependency, then he is able to become a real person for the patient, someone to develop an attachment to, learn to trust, and depend upon. The development of this dependency is necessary to compete with the obsessional defenses that were originally developed to compensate for failed dependency.

As for the therapist's fear of fostering this dependency on the part of his patients, it should be borne in mind that dependency that inadvertently develops within psychotherapy is ascribed to transference; therefore, the therapist is not manipulating the patient. Rather, he is letting the patient utilize the therapist as a screen upon which to project his or her feelings and ideas. The therapist need not feel responsible for the patient's attitude toward him or her.

If the therapist attempts to avoid this dependency—if, instead, he or she allows treatment to begin with the suggestion of a nondependent relationship—the patient will have his or her characteristic avoidance of dependency reinforced, thus fueling the drive to maintain his or her obsessional defenses. The patient already experiences a profound prohibition with regard to dependency and suffers from a premature pseudo-independence that has evolved into emotional isolation with symptomatic compensation. The self-soothing rituals, the repetitious thoughts, all serve to protect the patient from awareness of the need for comfort and support from another person. Therefore the beginning of treatment must explicitly state that the patient's resistance to dependency will be addressed by the therapist. This confrontation of the obsessional patient's resistance must begin during the initial interview in order to prevent the patient from establishing the therapy environment as new ground on which to employ obsessional defenses.

Actually, all forms of psychodynamic psychotherapy, with even the most passive of therapists, produce some degree of trust and dependency. What we are really discussing is whether this dependency must remain *implicit*—never dealt with or discussed—or *explicit*, identified and used by the therapist in deliberate structuring. Some therapists find dependency burdensome because it can lead to idealization and unrealistic demands for care and attention on the part of the patient. But this need not be true or, at least, does not have to create difficulty if the therapist takes the time to openly circumscribe the limits of the care allowed for in the therapeutic relationship. Most often, burdensome demands by a patient due to idealization occur because there is a difference in expectation between the two persons in the room.

For example, during a period of exceptional emotional stress for her, a patient anxiously told me, "I don't think seeing you three times a week is enough. I also wish that our sessions would go on all day and that I could go home with you at night."

I explained that her feelings were simply a wish that I were the all-loving parent she had always wanted. When she insisted that, whatever the reasons, she still wanted uninterrupted care and attention from me, it was necessary to confront her idealization.

"We have carefully constructed a helping environment here," I told her. "Part of what makes this helping environment succeed is the time limit on our sessions. If we had the open-ended session you propose, we would dilute the roles we have in terms of each other, and the structure that produces the kind of care you find so helpful would vanish."

She responded, "I still don't understand why you can't take me home with you."

"If I did that, I would soon find the level of care you request annoying, excessively demanding, and so I would find you a bother."

"Do you find me a bother now?"

"At this moment, I find you unrealistic, not wanting to understand the limits of care and therapy. I believe we will have made progress when you can understand those limits."

"But I'm not a bother now?"

"No, not as long as we stay within proper therapeutic borders."

While this patient had temporarily lost her sense of realistic limits, one of the major therapeutic issues here is the kind of countertransference her behavior might provoke in the therapist. One need not be frightened or repelled or discontinue treatment simply because the patient has idealized the therapist.

Several years ago, a colleague of mine was told by his patient that she was in love with him, and that she desired him sexually. He became very anxious and angrily exclaimed to her, "Why would I become sexually involved with you when I have a beautiful wife at home?" He promptly stopped treating the woman and referred her to another therapist.

It seems that transferences of idealization can be more difficult to cope with than transferences of hostility, which all therapists are so thoroughly trained to interpret. If the patient had professed hate instead of love, or the desire for murder instead of sex, my colleague would have been readily able to cope with the situation. This is doubly sad because fear of idealization can cause therapists to hinder its development (by being unnecessarily distant) during a patient's period of distress, and this can quickly lead to the end of meaningful treatment. With obsessional patients, a fear of abandonment by anyone they risk attachment to is the major impediment to the intensity of therapeutic engagement necessary to compensate for obsessional defenses.

NINE
Talking

With a nonobsessional patient, information gathering and personal and family history taking are important, not just in terms of the information delivered, but also because they assist the patient in talking to the therapist about nonthreatening subjects and, thereby, facilitate the gentle development of a benign transference. At least initially, the nonobsessional patient sees the therapist as a good listener, and the analytical or self-examination process is launched. This last aspect is most important since it is through the analytical process that the nonobsessional patient will confront repressed or denied feelings and understand why symptomatic attitudes and feelings develop. The very style of this relationship gives patients autonomy in the self-exploration process, implicity teaching them that they are responsible for therapeutic progress and, therefore, for the conduct of their lives.

In such treatment, it has been traditionally accepted that the patient does all, or at least 95 percent, of the talking in a psychotherapy session. But the empty OCD patient has very little to talk about and even less to analyze. A dwarfed sense of self, the absence of a language with which to think about one's self, the obsessive constriction that has minimized (over time) what reflective thoughts do occur to someone thinking in repetitious rituals, all can contribute to a near silent session.

Waiting the patient out with silence merely reinforces the theme of abandonment and is verification of the patient's feelings of inadequacy. Part of the therapist's nurturing is his or her talking to the patient. The silent patient is usually communicating nonverbally through facial gestures, muscle movements, postures, and other types of body language; mirroring this nonverbal but observable communication in a caring and interpretative way helps the therapist develop an alliance with the patient and fill the emptiness.

One technique taught to all therapists in training is to talk to the patient's strengths. But when working with obsessionally disordered patients, it becomes important to talk to the patient's emptiness. This cannot be done by assuring the patients they are not really empty and need only to find themselves. To obsessional ears, this says only that the therapist is unable to accept the truth of the emptiness or is unable to repair it.

If as a working definition of emptiness the patient's lack of mirroring and of parental identity messages is used, then compensating the patient means, first, accepting his or her emptiness; second, stating how the therapist expects to repair it; and third, talking sufficiently to develop transference to the point where the patient will be receptive to the therapist's mirroring. This will enable the patient to incorporate from the therapist's words appropriate identifying comments that, over the course of time in therapy, will help to clarify the sense of identity vagueness that the patient brings to the initial session.

Consider Dorothy, a fifteen-year-old who cannot find words to tell me about herself. She has been so reclusive in her lifestyle since the age of eleven that, even though she talks, she has no language to describe what she feels.

She became very anxious when I first suggested my need to know about her. "I can't talk about myself at all," she said in our initial meeting.

"Of course you can't," I told her. "Therapy is new to you.

Think of this. Suppose I said, 'Let's do therapy in French'? Then you'd say to me, 'I can't speak the language. We can't do therapy that way.' And I might answer, 'Well, I guess, first, I'll have to teach you how to speak French.' And so now I'm saying, before we start therapy, I have to teach you how to talk about yourself. Which means I'm going to have to talk about you for quite a while. And you'll remember what I say, and you'll learn to use my language to talk about yourself." Almost immediately, she was comfortable with the therapy.

Developmental deficits that prevent the patient from talking are often confused with resistance. For example, the very common therapist intervention, "How did you feel about that?" is often met with a sincere, "I don't know." If interpreted as resistance, this can be extremely frustrating to the therapist and may result in a very harmful power struggle between the two people in the room.

In the treatment of obsessional patients, the therapist must be ready and willing to talk endlessly, to fill the emptiness both in the room and in the patient, and to do this for a long period of time. Without such willingness, help would have been impossible for Nina, whom we met in chapter 4, a twelve-year-old girl who was psychotically withdrawn when I met her. For six months she had not eaten, drunk, or spoken a word. Previously hospitalized, she had been fed continuously by a nasogastric tube. At four feet nine, she weighed a deceptively normal eighty-four pounds due to the tube feeding. This small, fair, red-haired girl walked with robotlike movements, taking care to measure each step.

The psychiatrist treating Nina up to and during her previous hospitalization described the appearance of her symptoms: "By the time she had lost enough weight to require hospitalization, she had developed a peculiar speech pattern. Her voice became expressionless. The same thing happened to her gait, which became measured. She both walked and talked like a robot, and then she stopped speaking entirely. Her eating was ritualized; she drank out of measuring cups and beakers."

After a month of her first hospitalization, she had stopped

eating and drinking entirely and withdrawn beyond reach. Now, in her second hospitalization, Nina's ability to perform rituals had been severely restricted by the hospital staff. The clothing and toiletries that she arranged repeatedly were all removed from her room. (She could have any article she needed by asking a nurse for it; she was allowed to write out her requests.) Much of her day was spent in the hospital classroom where she did written work. The rest of her time was spent arranging and rearranging her clothing (after a written request for certain items). A pediatrician observing this endless, unself-conscious ritual—folding and refolding a garment with methodical precision—commented that it nearly brought tears to his eyes.

I met Nina during her first week of this second hospitalization. Her mother told me, in a resigned tone, "We have all but given up hope and understand that she may die. But we just wanted you to see if there's anything you could do."

At our first meeting, Nina walked the length of the adolescent medicine office in a measured pace, staring straight ahead. Her head unswervingly faced the direction in which she was walking. I directed her to sit down, wondering what I was going to do with a patient who had not spoken for six months. Waiting in silence for Nina to speak first would've been out of the question. I would have to talk to her until she could begin to answer. I would aim to interpret her silence, infer as much as possible, and state the inference as if it were a response to her spoken words.

"Hello, Nina."

She nodded, with a blank expression, but her eyes were focused.

I assumed she was receptive regardless of her response. "I believe you would like to get rid of what prevents you from talking, eating, and drinking," I suggested. "Also, you probably wish you didn't have to be so careful of the way you do everything . . . like folding your clothing so often."

She said nothing, but I inferred agreement.

"Well then," I continued, "the first thing I need to explain to you is why people try to be so desperately careful, the way you do."

She made eye contact and held it.

I went on for a half hour, maintaining as much eye contact as she could reciprocate as I explained to her that rituals are procedures that create a kind of security and that people who use them have a hard time trusting others, as well as themselves. At this point, Nina began to cry. At first she was inaudible, then her crying became voiced, as if she were saying no in protest to what I was saying. I stopped and offered her tissues to wipe her nose.

I asked her, "Do you have a hard time trusting yourself?"

She continued to cry in protest while making intense eye contact.

"Are you able to feel secure when you are at home? Do you wonder about how much people care about you?"

Nina's crying became so intense at this point that we both became preoccupied with getting enough tissues to deal with her profusely running nose, and I untangled the hyperalimentation line that stretched from her chest to the infusion pump. (She had wound it around her arm.) Eventually Nina stopped crying but maintained eye contact.

Nina and other patients who are similarly withdrawn are difficult to work with because they tend to offer the therapist so little in the way of information and behavior. Silence as a provocative device fails. Talking to a nonresponsive patient is taxing, and the patient's silence may produce anger in the therapist. After all, isn't he doing all the work (talking)? The therapist begins to resent the patient and may shift in his own feelings from trying to cajole the patient into talking, to imploring and even threatening the patient into talking. A statement sometimes made (in frustration) to nontalking inpatients in psychiatric hospitals by beginning psychiatrists is, "You know, I get paid whether you get better or not." This is harmful to the patient and is indicative of inadequate training.

Nina's long-term silence, along with her measured gait and other compulsive behavior, suggested a fear of talking imperfectly. This proved to be a useful interpretation in that it drew more crying from Nina. She did not attempt to leave the room or even look away from me. This voiced crying became Nina's sole mode of expression for six weeks. Coping with her running nose became additional behavior between therapist and patient. Physical clinging to the therapist became a verification of positive contact. For six weeks, then, I talked for most of each session as if responding to Nina's words. Areas I discussed included fears of inadequacy, abandonment, failure, disapproval by others, and distrust of self, as well as fears about being let down by others. I spoke in each area, first by using the generalized "one," then by illustrating with her own case.

After six weeks of my talking, she broke her silence. A nurse passing Nina in the hallway said her usual, "Good morning, Nina. How are you?" Over her shoulder, she heard a wooden, strained, measured, "I . . . am . . . fine . . . thank . . . you."

Her talking was a major breakthrough; she had been silent for many months. After several more weeks, the stiffness of her speech began to fade, although she was still performing most tasks in a ritualistic manner. For instance, Nina was offered beakers and containers of bottled water from which she could drink. It was preferable to allow her to begin drinking in this manner, which she found agreeable, than to continue her intravenous feeding indefinitely. By bringing her the water and giving her the beakers, I now had a part in her ritualized behavior pattern, and, therefore, would soon be able to modify it.

These therapy sessions with Nina consisted of my talking to her and looking for nonverbal verification or rejection of what I had just said. Each day I would prepare a topic, one that represented an adolescent concern and could be seen as partially contributing to the severe withdrawal and the use of obsessive-compulsive defenses we were seeing. I had no expectations for responses on her part, and this protected me from experiencing hostile feelings that Nina was withholding communication. Instead, I conveyed to her that I felt she would be unable to make verbal responses for some time to come. I told her that until she was able to talk to me, I would talk to her. I believe that she then experienced my speaking to her as my taking care of her. After seven weeks of therapy, she began to come out of her severe withdrawal. First she risked drinking water. Then she began to eat. It took more than a year for her to relinquish her severe way of eating in which she used six plates, eventually modifying it to two three-section plates before finally giving them up for one plate.

Throughout this period no medication was used. Several months after hospital discharge, Nina left treatment. Her mother continued to talk with me about strategies to further reduce Nina's obsessive-compulsive behavior. Upon follow-up two years later with the pediatrician, Nina was reported as displaying no remarkable psychological symptoms.

What is particularly unusual about Nina's case is that a minimum of background information was presented. When treatment began, of course, Nina could not speak, and her family would not or could not present more than the barest outline about her past. And when Nina's most obvious obsessional symptoms had disappeared, her family could not be persuaded to continue psychotherapy.

What we do know is that the family experienced the loss of an infant due to crib death only one year before Nina became ill, and that Nina overheard her mother's comment, "Oh dear, she's dead." But we have no way of knowing how this affected Nina.

She had an older sister and a younger brother, both still living, and both parents, still married. So except for the baby's death, her family was intact. But there was no other information about exceptional situations in the family relationships.

Yet without vital information or thoughts from the patient herself, I had to continue with treatment based on almost nothing other than the behavioral symptoms with which I was coping. With only this, a remarkable recovery was achieved based solely on one kind of behavior (treatment) on my part.

That behavior apparently worked with minimal input from family and patient.

This offers some clear indications about the uniformity of deprivation that can cause OCD, and it says that sometimes OCD can be treated blindly, even when knowing almost nothing about the patient's or family background, and being aware of only the most basic dynamics involved in the development of the disorder.

TEN
The New Therapy

If OCD is viewed as a set of behaviors and thoughts evolved by individuals as a way of coping with anxiety that arose out of a failure of dependency, then the need for these people to utilize dependency—to learn how to depend on another person—to relieve those self-propelled rituals can also be seen. Patients themselves sometimes recognize this need, although their words may not be the same.

When thirty-year-old Annabelle, whom we also met in chapter 4, came to me, she said at once that she needed a caring therapist. She had been in treatment twice before but felt that both of the therapists had not really cared about her. In effect, she represented herself as a person in need of someone powerful enough for her to invest with her dependency. On some level, she knew this was where her other therapists had failed.

Nineteen-year-old Katharine, too, whom we've also met, was able to make this need clear. "I was in analysis before I went to college and after I left," she told me in our first meeting. "But nothing ever happens. I feel like I could go to Dr. B. forever and nothing will change. I go there; he waits for me to talk. I begin to talk about things, and I feel like I'm at confession with a priest, except Dr. B. never blesses me, and I don't know if he thinks I should be forgiven."

"Forgiven for what?"

"For having no life," she explained. "For moving away from everyone I know. For making rituals my whole life. I don't know what was supposed to happen with Dr. B. He was a nice man; he was polite. But I never knew what he thought about anything I said. I just felt alone in the room, waiting for something to happen that would change everything. But nothing ever happened. I just talked."

Clearly, a more participating therapist was needed if Katharine was to be helped. As a young child growing up in an affluent family, Katharine had been raised and attended to by a nanny. What she could observe of her parents' relationship was a father sexually interested in her mother in a dominant, almost abusive, and indiscreet manner. He often made Katharine feel embarrassed. He was critical of Katharine's shortcomings: of any grade less than an A, of her hair for being too curly, of the amount of makeup she wanted to use. What was absent from their relationship was any positive expression about her on his part. She only remembers one compliment.

"The night he killed himself, he told me I was beautiful."

Katharine was fourteen when her father committed suicide. She was sixteen when the nanny who had taken care of her since the age of four died of a stroke.

When Katharine came to me, she had been in psychoanalysis for three years (with Dr. B.) for withdrawing into depression, characterized by obsessive-compulsive behavior (excessive cleanliness, exercising, orderliness, and compulsive reading of newspapers and magazines), and then anorexia nervosa, which intensified her ritualized patterns. Finally, she had been hospitalized for emaciation. The diagnosis at the New York City teaching hospital was "Borderline Personality Disorder, Prognosis: fair." She left the hospital after six months, having nearly achieved her goal weight. But several months later, her weight had dropped again, down to eighty-two pounds (she was five feet six).

In that first interview, I asked her, "Who else do you talk to aside from Dr. B.?"

"I don't have time for that. I talk to my mother, who lives in another state with my—with her husband. They just got married. But when my friends call, I just tell them I'm busy and will have to call them back . . . which I never do. I have too many rituals to be bothered." Abruptly, she looked around the room at the paintings on the walls. "Who did the paintings?" she asked.

"My wife . . . except for the Wyeth print."

"I like them." She smiled nervously.

"Why are you here?" I asked her. "What can I do for you?"

"I don't know what you can do for me, but I'm here because I have no life."

"What does that mean?"

She was torn between needing to portray herself as relaxed and sociable, and the desire to express all of her pent-up energy. She chose a calm narrative style, as if she were explaining the plight of someone else in her family.

"I live alone," she said, "and I do nothing but rituals all day. It wasn't like that before I went into the hospital, but it's been that way ever since I came out. I've lost touch with my high-school friends who are now in college. I never made friends in college, the one year I was there. And I don't have time for any friends now."

"So it's been rituals instead of people, and yet you're coming to a person—to me—to stop you from doing them?"

"I don't know that it's rituals instead of people. When I was in high school, it *was* people. I had friends . . . and boyfriends. But it's been like this for three years, and it's getting worse."

"What happened while you were in high school?"

"My father died when I was fourteen. He killed himself."

"Did all this begin then?"

"No. It began two years later, when Anna died."

"Who is Anna?"

"Anna was my . . . well, you would have to call her a nanny. She took care of my brother and me. She took care of us more than anyone else."

"More than your parents?"

"More than anybody." She became tearful.

"Who has taken care of you since then?" I asked.

"I was sixteen. No one needs to be taken care of at that age."

"And what about now? Don't you need to be taken care of now?"

Openly crying, she told me, "I'm nineteen. I should be able to take care of myself."

"But you're not able to."

"What do you mean?" The tears suddenly halted, replaced by angry protest. "I completely take care of myself now. I live alone. I do everything for myself."

"You live a ritual-ridden existence. You're a skeleton, so we know that you can't feed yourself successfully. Your ritual schedule doesn't allow you to go to school or go to work or see friends. It seems to me that you need lots of care."

"I thought you were supposed to make me feel better. Isn't that why you get paid?"

"Do you always become contemptuously tyrannical when you're frightened?"

"Therapists are supposed to make people feel better, aren't they?"

"You pay me, as you put it, to make decisions about how to cope with you in such a way as to help you overcome your problems. Even though you pay me, I remain in charge of what happens in this room. Even though this is an office, what happens here happens between two real people, and, hopefully, it will help you change in a way that will help you overcome your problems."

"Dr. B. would never talk to me like that."

"You mean he would never tell you if you were acting out?"

"You can't accuse me of things! You're my therapist!"

As shocked and upset as she sounded, I knew that my attitude had accomplished its purpose: Katharine had become engaged in treatment. As the interview continued, she managed to give me significant historical material but, more importantly, she presented her own psychodynamic history as well. She indicated that she could not further benefit from analytical inquiry at this point in her life. She left treatment with an analyst of fine repute. It was the style of treatment she had rejected, not the particular analyst. A supervising analyst might argue that it was her resistance to threatening issues that caused her premature termination. But in all likelihood, it was her emptiness that made her inadequate to utilize psychoanalytic psychotherapy.

Katharine's father's suicide, her being raised by a nanny, all suggested to her than she was not worth caring for, or was too much of a burden for her parents. Any mode of therapy that placed responsibility on her would be experienced as another form of abandonment. The therapist who conducted such a therapy with her would be viewed as dependent upon her for success. Her own transferential expectations were that I would be weak and, thus, contemptible. She required reassurance that I was not abandoning and dependent.

Her anxiety level was raised when I addressed the issue of the forbidden wish—her need for care. Her challenging behavior was an attempt to discourage me from pursuing a caring role with her in order for her to keep her defensive denial intact. It was her defensive denial that fueled her obsessive-compulsive disorder as well as her anorexia nervosa.

Several months after our initial session, it became apparent that Katharine would require a second hospitalization due to continued low weight coupled with strenuous, compulsive exercise. This time a medical hospital was selected. Three weeks prior to hospitalization, I discussed my plan with her.

"You know I hate hospitals," she told me, partially angry, partially resigned.

"And because I'm aware of that, we'll use a medical hospital. It won't be to cure you, just to recover your weight, which is dangerously low."

She seemed more conciliatory. "Part of me knows that I

should gain weight. But part of me is irrational about it and knows if I'm left to my own devices, I'll never do it." She paused, then said slowly, "The scariest part of going into a hospital is not the weight gain, it's losing control over . . . well, you know, over my rituals." She had been staring at the floor, but now she looked up. "I know that I'm weird. But even though I know that, the weird things that I do—they are very, very important to me."

"I guess you'll have to compromise about this."

"That's easy for you to say. You're not jeopardizing your whole security system!"

"But the fact that you're aware of why you need the rituals—as a security system—that should make it easier for you to distance yourself a bit from the compulsion to act on it."

She looked at me as if I were an idiot and, half condescending, half trapped, said, "No. Somehow it doesn't work that way. Whether it's about eating and weight, or whether it's about all the other rituals, there never seems to be much choice about doing them."

"Does it seem like there are specific consequences if you *don't* do them?"

She shrugged her shoulders and returned her gaze to the carpet, her knuckles whitening as she clenched her fists. She took a deep breath, exhaled, unfolded her fingers and stared at her nails to regain composure. "No," she said, "there are no particular consequences I envision if I fail to do my special behavior. There are no thoughts about what will happen to me. There are feelings of intense dread, however, and these feelings are so strong that to invite them in by failing to do behaviors is unthinkable. So you see, it's not a free choice. It's not a decision-making process. I guess that's why everybody calls them compulsions."

She seemed assertive while explaining this to me, more so than at any other time in her treatment. And it became clear to me that at this point the illness itself had become her basis for assertiveness. Without it, she might feel that she had no assertiveness. And that would be another kind of loss for her.

My words were chosen carefully. "I appreciate the intensity of your anxiety, your pain, and even panic about having to give up the privacy to do that which you are compelled to do. If your health and safety weren't involved, we would have more choice. But we don't. For medical reasons we are forced to hospitalize you and externally restrict your privacy to prevent you from performing these security-making rituals."

She feigned annoyance, but it was more despair that showed on her face. "It's easy for you to say. You don't have to do it."

"I never lose sight of that. But I still have to say it, and you still have to do it."

"Does this mean that you're getting rid of me?"

"No. It means that I will have to see you at the hospital, and I'll have to talk to doctors and nurses about you several times a week."

She looked surprised and relieved, but then a new light came into her eyes. "What will you tell them?"

I smiled. "I'll tell them how to be as mean to you as I am, of course."

"No, really. What will you say to them about me?"

"I will tell them about your problems, your symptoms, some family background so that they can understand you and be sensitive to your needs. They won't necessarily do what you want them to do. But they will do what should be done."

"What does that mean?"

"It means you'll lose your privacy, and you'll lose your control over your weight."

"And when I lose my privacy, it will be much harder for me to do the special things I need to do."

"That will be harder for you to tolerate than your weight gain?"

"Oh yes. I don't know if I can."

"You'll have to."

She shook her head. "I don't know if I like this whole idea. I don't know if I can do it."

"Of course you don't like this, but you have to do it. There's no choice."

"Don't sound so bossy. You're not my mother, you know."

"Your mother's not this bossy."

"You sound like all of this is finalized."

I nodded. "I've put in a call to get you a bed at the beginning of next week."

"Oh shit! You aren't kidding."

"Nope."

Katharine's medical hospitalization took place as scheduled. She managed to salvage most of her obsessive-compulsive behaviors, minus her weight and eating control. The hospital staff required that I be "bad cop" as well as psychotherapist in order to ensure her compliance with medical-surgical feeding protocol. This provided many opportunities to deepen transference and attachment, and for us to examine what was happening between us. In an inpatient setting such as this, the therapist is part of a team. It is a situation that invites vulnerability for the therapist because he has "real life" authority over the patient. The therapist's reactions to the patient, and to her treatment, can provide countertransferential pitfalls.

During her hospitalization, Katharine was refed by a catheter placed in her jugular vein that required some surgery to implant. I attended the surgical procedure and talked her through it. I explained each step to her, much to the surgeon's delight, because he felt this made her more cooperative than most patients. The nutritional fluids began to flow; Katharine was passive about her weight gain. When she became upset about any aspect of her hospitalization, she would vent her unhappiness at me. That was fine. During her struggle with her weight and eating obsessions, and through her displacing that struggle partially onto me, she began to incorporate my values for her appearance and weight. By the time Katharine was ready for discharge from the hospital, her protests about her new appearance were mild.

Katharine was, however, as ritual-ridden as ever, and her social life was nonexistent. My attempts to encourage her to contact old friends were met with anger and protests. For a period in Katharine's therapy, she was responding to me often with anger and contempt. One day I remarked to her, "I have something to teach you."

She cut me off with, "You have *nothing* to teach me."

As in the beginning of her therapy, I felt that I had to overcome her contempt with an explicit assertiveness of my own. My response to her comment was, "I have a lot to teach you, and you have to learn from me."

She then said a very touching thing to me. Looking both frustrated and frightened, she said softly, "Do you know that you're the only person I talk to during the day about anything personal?"

In her own way, she was telling me how frightening it was to fight or argue with me. She was like an early adolescent, and she had the needs of one, such as arguing with a parent. But she did not have the security to argue without reassurance that she would not be abandoned. Abandonment was a major theme in her life.

I reminded her of something I had said previously to her. "What goes on in this room is primarily my responsibility. If we have to struggle because that's important to do at this point, then that's what we'll do. You don't have to worry that I will throw you out if you say the wrong thing here. I assume that we will work through all our disagreements, and I consider you my problem. I wouldn't have it any other way."

She laughed with relief. "Well, lucky you."

Katharine's statement, "You have nothing to teach me!" was her attempt to devalue me and thereby calm her fears of depending on me as a teacher. Rather than present that interpretation to her at the time, I chose to self-confidently maintain that I was indeed the teacher. In doing this, I deepened the ambivalence and, therefore, the attachment. When Katharine accused me of being bossy and reminded me that I was not her mother, I explained that her mother was not bossy. In fact, bossy people were more attractive to her.

One day in session, I noticed that Katharine's posture changed toward me from straightforward and friendly to haughty and cold. We had just been talking about her changeability about men, and she was saying, "It seems that if I like a man, he's usually disinterested in me. If I can get him interested in me, I'm no longer interested in him."

"I have noticed here that if I'm solicitous of you, you become distant and disinterested in our conversation."

"I've noticed the same thing. Sometimes I just disconnect."

"Yet if I shift my tone to a more demanding one, even a harsh tone, you become much more pleasant. Instead of being afraid of a stronger tone from me, you seem to like it better. What do you think your attraction to that stronger posture is?"

She looked embarrassed, shrugged her shoulders, and smiled. "Do you think that I'm masochistic or something?"

"I think it's more complicated than that. You seem to equate thoughtfulness and sensitivity toward you with weakness. You perhaps equate harshness and criticalness with strength. I wonder who taught you that these traits and behaviors go together?"

She began haltingly, "My father never gave me a compliment. He looked at my report card and asked me about the only B but never mentioned all the As. He told me that my hair was too curly, so I've ironed it since I was eight years old." She became tearful. "I only wish he were still alive so he could see what I've done and what I'll be able to do. He only knew this inadequate little girl."

"I guess it was really important to finally win him over, to finally get some praise from him."

"I'm not sure praise and Daddy are in the same universe."

"I guess if I sound critical or harsh, it makes you feel like I'm worth winning over."

She nodded her head. "Then you sound like a Daddy person."

"If I sound nice or soft, who does that sound like?"

"I guess then maybe you're a Mommy person."

"Is it good to be a Mommy person?"

"Mommy person is always criticized by Daddy person, unless he's fooling around with her."

"What do you mean?"

"You know, romantically. He really liked her 'that way.'"

"Do you feel that the only way he appreciated her was romantically?"

"It seemed so."

"Was it hard for you to get your mother's approval?"

"It was easy, and she was never critical. But somehow, when she complimented me, it didn't work. It's not that I didn't believe her. I believed that she meant what she said, but I guess I couldn't value it much."

"Then just the granting of a compliment from a person makes them seem weak or devalued to you?"

"I guess so. Does that mean I'll never be able to have a relationship with a man? It's what I've always feared."

"We can use our therapy as a workshop to change your associations. You have the same reactions to me. When I'm nice, I seem like your mother, and you become contemptuous. And when I'm confrontational or critical, you attribute more prestige and esteem to me. That gives us a way to work on the problem. It may take a long time, but I believe we can change a good deal of that."

Here I was reinforcing the therapeutic prescription of attachment. Katharine's questioning was an indication of attachment and trust. When she asked about herself she was letting me know she might be able to incorporate the answers I gave her. Once she could use her attachment to me to incorporate new ideas about herself, then this process would compete with the one of being obsessionally critical of herself. In other words, she would replace her obsessional, critical voice with that of the therapist, thereby giving up her obsessional system for an interpersonal one. In order to do this, she had to become extremely trusting and attached.

I would continue to use this attachment to break into the obsessional system and the mental and emotional inertia it maintained. I would also use guidance, advice, and teaching to clarify the confusion and compensate for the deficits that years of obsessional stagnation had produced.

ELEVEN
Family Therapy

Individuals suffering from obsessional disorders are often raised by exhausted, depleted parents who are themselves needy. Now if you are reading this book as a parent, and you are not at least partially exhausted and drained as a result of your childraising responsibilities along with all your other tasks, then clearly someone else is bringing up your children. But there is a qualitative distinction between parents who are occasionally worn out and parents who are so used up by their work lives or health problems or other emotional disturbances that they communicate to the child that they would prefer for nurturance to run the other way. These are the depleted parents I speak about: those who typically communicate neediness, a reversal of power, and an implicit reversal of dependency with that child; those who do this to such an extent that the child is construed as the more powerful and the parent is looked upon as the one in need.

Often this situation is characterized by parents deferring to their children, asking their offspring to make premature choices. When a parent asks a five-year-old where he or she would like to go on vacation, this is clearly a premature choice.

When a six-year-old is asked what elementary school that child would care to attend, this is another example. Even parents asking an eight-year-old which restaurant to go to is a premature choice. So the indicators of this role and power reversal are the offering of inappropriate decisions to a young child, the constant deferring to the child, the consistent requesting of approval from the child.

When this theme exists between parents and one of their children, then that child is, in effect, parentified. This parentification is an abandonment of the child and teaches him that no one is there to help, guide, or protect him.

The compensatory role for the psychotherapist is to fill this nurturing vacuum. But there are actually two vacuums to be filled: the absence of support that both the child and the parents are experiencing. Unless these needs are treated simultaneously, success in changing the child's obsessional behavior is not likely. But this demands full-family therapy, and there are major problems with conventional family therapy in the treatment of obsessional disorders. This is clearly illustrated by the case of Rebecca and her parents.

Rebecca was sixteen and the youngest of three children. Her two older brothers were in their late twenties. One was a lawyer; the other was struggling to establish himself in the sales division of a large corporation. Both brothers lived at home with Rebecca and their parents. Her mother found their living arrangement acceptable since they had a large house and the sons made no demand on family income. The father, however, was constantly irritated by the boys' presence.

Over a three-year period, Rebecca had developed an increasing pattern of obsessive-compulsive disorders. Her rituals had multiplied to the point where she had drifted off from her friends and was unable to get her schoolwork done on time because she was preoccupied with the many rituals she had to complete before beginning her homework each night. The more apparent her rituals became to her family, the more angered they became. Her brothers had taken to calling her crazy, at first out of her presence, but later to her directly. She had taken to isolating herself in her room. They noticed that she would touch doorknobs only while holding a tissue or napkin. They also noticed that she had developed a peculiar pattern of walking around carefully in her room, as if she were trying to avoid stepping on objects only she could see.

After a few sessions alone with Rebecca, I asked the other members of the family to come in together for an evaluation. They sat in two clusters. Rebecca sat down first, and her mother sat next to her. The brothers sat across from Rebecca, and their father, after staring awkwardly at the two groups for several moments, sat next to the boys.

The mother spoke first. "We're quite concerned about Rebecca. She seems to be withdrawing from all of us and from the rest of her life at an increasing rate. I know that she's been seeing you in therapy, and I'm afraid that she would not tell you everything that she's doing or having trouble with."

Rebecca remained expressionless, as if in a trance.

Andrew (the middle child) took over. "I'm worried, too. It's like Rebecca just keeps getting weirder all the time. She fusses with everything. She examines her clothing as if something terrible might be on it. I mean, she looks each skirt or blouse—even her socks—over like there might be a bug in them that she'd better get off or it will kill her or something. She showers for hours, At least it seems like hours."

The older brother, Harvey, spoke then. In contrast to Andrew, his pace and intensity were slower and more relaxed. "We just think she's getting harder to reach," he told me. "When she was a little kid . . ." He became a bit tearful. ". . . she used to want to talk to me all the time. Most of the time I didn't even have the time to talk to her. But some of the time I did. She was always such a fun kid. She always had a million questions. She really loved it when I talked to her. I could always tell that. Now, she's like a ghost who stalks the house." Harvey turned toward Rebecca. "See how she looks now? Expressionless. That's how she looks most of the time. I wish we . . . I could get her back. It's like she's gone." Recovering his composure, he asked, "Is there something we can do to get her well? Sometimes I just want to grab her and shake her and yell at her to cut out all that weird stuff."

After the two brothers spoke, the room became silent. I attempted to shift the focus. "There are still two people we haven't heard from. Would either of them like to speak?"

Rebecca remained silent and expressionless, as if she had not heard me.

Her father rubbed the top of his head as if searching for something to offer. Finally, he said, "I don't know. I just don't know." He turned to Rebecca. "How can we help you, honey? Is there something you need from us that you're not getting? We need your input here. I would like to know how you would like us to help you."

Now Rebecca became tearful. She fended off crying as intensely as she could, which made the first burst of tears come out in a rush and a rage. "I just wish you could be a real father!"

"What do you mean?" he asked defensively.

"Why are you always asking me what to do? If I knew what to do, I wouldn't need you!" Her crying overwhelmed her for a minute. The family remained silent. Finally Rebecca continued. "A real father knows what to do. He doesn't ask his kid what to do."

"Rebecca, I am your real father."

"It just doesn't feel like it." She became expressionless and silent again.

Her father turned to me for support; held out his hands, palms up, and shrugged his shoulders. Rebecca's mother rolled her eyes in exasperation, as if agreeing with her daughter. Her brothers looked at each other and shook their heads.

"What are you feeling?" I asked the brothers.

Harvey answered. "I don't know if this has ever happened before; that is, if we have ever said the same things to each other before, but this all feels very familiar. I feel like we're cursed or something, forced to repeat this hopeless exercise again and again. It just doesn't feel like there's anything new happening here."

* * *

In my next individual meeting with Rebecca, I asked her about the family session. "How did you feel about your brothers and your parents?"

"I feel like they did what they wanted to. They told on me. They came here, and they cleaned up their act so they wouldn't sound as mean and crummy as they do at home, so they could find more polite ways to tell me how crazy I am."

"When your father asked you what he could do for you, why did you get so upset?"

"Because he's useless to my mother. I don't know which makes me angrier, when he's a jerk with me or when he's useless to her."

"How do you know that he's useless to her?"

"He's never affectionate to her. He's never thoughtful about her feelings. He's as bad a husband as he is a father."

"Are you angry for yourself or for your mother?"

"Both."

Rather than work with all members of the family together (as would be done in conventional family therapy), I elected to refer Rebecca's parents for couples therapy, in order for them to explore their relationship and their parenting of Rebecca. The therapist who would work with them would have two goals: to develop a supportive role with them, in effect, to nurture them; and, at the same time, to teach them more role-appropriate parenting with their daughter, taking a more maternal and paternal role with their daughter, treating her as if she were younger.

They would be instructed to view her obsessive-compulsive defenses as her way of trying to control her anxieties and her fears, and to react to her as if she were a child in distress who needs guidance, structuring, and affection. They would be warned that she would refuse this support for quite a while, but that they must continue to offer her these postures nonetheless.

The rationale for separating the family of an obsessive-compulsive individual into the two therapy units is that in sessions together, the parents would continue to complain about their daughter, and the therapist's attempts at corrective behavior (made in full view of the daughter) would implicitly prove to her that her parents were weak and that she was unprotected by them as well as unguided by them. She would see her parents as circumstantially demeaned by the therapist, and their own neediness might just continue to emerge, deepening the dysfunctional roles they played with her.

I told Rebecca that her parents should have their own therapist, working only with them, while she would continue to have her own, too. I was also indicating implicitly that there would be nurturance added to the family system on two levels, so that she would no longer be needed as her mother's nurturer or as the detractor during spouse conflict. Her response to the recommendations was simply, "I hope they'll do it."

A major goal in redirecting parents of obsessionally disordered children and adolescents is to develop in them a posture of constructive interference. In the past, the prescription of the individual psychotherapist for the parents was often: "Give the child more space; don't be intrusive." What these recommendations did was to further disenfranchise parents who already suffered from a lack of self-confidence about their role as parents. Rebecca's father characterized this when he asked her, "How would you like us to help you?" Helping a parent restructure the family system is not the role of the patient. It is the role of the therapist.

Unfortunately, not all therapists recognize the important part parents can play in treating the obsessional individual. Some consider that parental participation should consist solely in delivering the patient to the therapist's office and then getting her home. This was the case with the first therapist who treated twelve-year-old Lara, who took on the role of nurturer to her mother at a very early age (previously discussed). At the end of each session, the therapist would walk Lara to the door and smilingly reassure her parents, "Everything is all right."

"But everything was certainly not all right," Lara informed

me in our initial meeting. "That's why I repeatedly told my parents that therapy was a waste of time."

I explained to Lara that I would have to help her grow up; that she might need to see me until she became eighteen and left for college, and that I would also recommend therapy for her parents.

I had Lara's parents enter therapy with a co-therapist whose task it was to assist them in analyzing those aspects of the family system that fostered or perpetuated Lara's symptoms. They were instructed to set limits to reduce Lara's acting-out behavior. In the past, Lara had exhibited temper tantrums that were characterized by her screaming until she was exhausted. Now, when this began to happen, Lara's mother made reassuring statements about her affection for Lara, but at the same time forbade her to act frenzied. In addition, Lara was referred to a psychopharmacologist for evaluation. He prescribed a benzodiazepine for panic attacks. The intensity, though not the frequency, of her panic attacks diminished.

Thanks to the separate therapy, Lara's mother became assertive in the feeding of her daughter. For a period of time she actually spoon-fed her, and Lara gained fifteen pounds in eight weeks.

At first Lara's father seemed overwhelmed by his daughter's ritualistic behaviors and angry tantrums. He often expressed doubts about her recovery to the family therapist and admitted that he could not cope with Lara the way his wife did. This presented the opportunity in the couple's sessions to explore their long-standing resentments toward each other. Chief among them was each spouse's feeling that the other was not appreciative. The father felt that he sacrificed enormous amounts of time and energy to provide well for his family, and he was angry that his wife never acknowledged that he had done it all for them. His wife felt emotionally abandoned by her husband's singular devotion to his work, and she felt that he belittled the job she had to do as a virtual single parent.

Lara's identification with her mother made her feel abandoned and angry. She clung to her mother and punished her father with distance and illness. Indeed, Lara felt overly dependent on her only at-home parent; during each of her therapy sessions, she had to walk out to the waiting room once or twice to make certain her mother was still there. It would take two years, but Lara's mother was finally able to leave the waiting room without Lara, experiencing a panic attack. It is doubtful that this could have been achieved without separate therapy for the parents as well as for the patient.

In the unusual case of Emily, the family did not wait for their daughter's rituals to become set in concrete before a therapist was contacted. Emily was eight years old when she began to act "peculiar," according to her mother. A few years later she had undergone a medical diagnostic work-up for gastrointestinal distress. The diagnosis was negative, and Emily's distress was labeled idiopathic. A month after the diagnostic examinations, Emily began to worry about her food causing more distress. She asked her mother for reassurances that she would not be made sick by meals served to her. She was given many assurances by her mother, but her requests seemed to increase daily.

Mealtime became a dreaded situation for the family as Emily demanded to know how carefully the silverware had been washed and how clean the table was. Her parents entered therapy for assistance in coping with their daughter, as well as for their own feelings of fright and anger over her behavior. They expressed their fear that she might permanently be a sick person. They were concerned about the extremely high level of anxiety that Emily was experiencing and her increasingly phobic behavior. Despite their best efforts, Emily could not be comforted or reassured adequately. They needed a strategy that would reduce her fear of being poisoned and the accompanying cleanliness rituals they were seeing.

Had her parents complied with the child's persistent pleas to clean and reclean all food-related items, they would have been reenforcing an obsessive safety system and acknowledging that this was a more powerful source of comfort. They used the therapist's advice as support for the difficult task of resisting Emily's orders.

What evolved was a strategy of parental noncompliance with regard to Emily's unreasonable demands for reassurance or for any additional cleaning of dishes, silverware, or the table. Emily was told that if she had doubts about the cleanliness of these items, she would have to wash them herself, and that her parents disapproved of additional cleaning.

For several weeks, Emily became increasingly adamant in her demands. Her parents responded calmly and did not comply. Over a period of six weeks, Emily's anxiety peaked. She had tantrums, screamed at her parents night and day, and demanded that objects around her be washed. At one point, the parents wondered if Emily could be controlled and if they could continue to care for her at home. But by the eighth week of this ongoing battle, it was clear that Emily's energy and intensity was diminishing from what appeared to be a phobic to a moderately anxious level.

It was three years before Emily stopped questioning sanitary issues beyond a reasonable point. The continual diminishing of her intensity about it helped support her parents' program of noncompliance with her unreasonable requests. Throughout this period, the assertive noncompliance on the part of Emily's parents provoked an important conflict in the patient. The obsessional system she was developing would have completely separated her (making her emotionally inaccessible) and ultimately disenfranchised her parents. Had this happened, Emily's system would have remained intact, perhaps throughout her lifetime, her inaccessibility deepening as time went on.

Since her parents were able to interfere with Emily's system at the onset (or at least its observable onset), Emily was forced to choose between her parents' judgments and the self-soothing system she was attempting to withdraw into. Her parents' assertiveness made the system weaker in that it could not dominate the family. At the same time, her parents' interference caused Emily to experience them as sturdier, more reliable, and therefore more attractive than the system.

Emily's tantrums during this period represented the conflict she was engaged in: whether to remain attached to her parents and to use them as guiding and supportive people, or whether to detach from them and form multiple obsessive-compulsive rituals to, in effect, take her parents' place. Since we assume that this struggle was unconscious on Emily's part, she would not welcome but rather resist her parents' demands that she change her behavior. She would not reward them for trying to make her a healthier person. This made matters more difficult for her parents. As Emily became more anxious, their natural inclination was to lower her level of anxiety by complying with her wishes, rather than to raise it with more noncompliant behavior. It was the support they received from the therapist that enabled them to continually interfere with the OCD system's growth and utilization by Emily.

On a six-year follow-up, Emily showed no signs of OCD, was a well-adjusted high school student, and her parents' therapist reported that Emily herself has never been in therapy. When she experienced anxiety, she was able to talk with her parents, air her feelings, and feel better. Her parents' resourcefulness ultimately made them more attractive to this anxious child than the obsessive-compulsive system she was attempting to develop.

Emily's problem was probably two-fold. In the first instance, she was always perceived as a rather anxious child; her parents coped with her anxiety by deferring to her or giving in to her, fearful of her throwing tantrums or becoming even more worrisome. Emily understood her parents' giving in as meaning she was in charge. This merely worsened her anxiety.

Trauma came when Emily was diagnosed as possibly having some gastrointestinal problem. She mistakenly saw her parents' words and actions as abandonment. They took her to the hospital, "surrendered" her to the doctors for tests, and made comments about the doctors being in charge and responsible for decisions about Emily's future. This greatly exacerbated Emily's normal anxiety. She began to believe that her parents were defeated by her personality (and its anxiety) and by some mysterious medical condition for which she was turned over to the care of doctors.

Very often in pediatric medicine children can misunderstand being cared for by a physician, especially if it involves hospitalization or unpleasant and frightening tests. The child may perceive the parents' helplessness in the face of a possible illness as a sign of abandonment, and if the child has anxiety to begin with, he or she may now try to replace the parents with obsessional defenses.

Children often come down with obsessional and eating disorders after a period of hospitalization and examination. Obviously, special attention must be paid to the way medical care is offered to children so that misunderstanding is avoided. Children should not be allowed to feel they are ill because of parental failure, and they should not be permitted to feel that their parents are surrendering them to doctors. It must be indicated to children that the medical profession is assisting parents in their nurturing, and the posture must be a collaborative effort between parents and physicians.

TWELVE
Prognosis

In any discussion of chronic psychological disorders, questions always arise about prognosis, or outlook for the future. The most frequent question I hear about obsessive-compulsive disorders is "Does anyone ever become cured, or is one always in a stage of recovery, facing a permanent danger of relapse?" (As one is always an alcoholic, according to the prevailing opinions about alcoholism.)

Prognosis varies with the mental health of the individual. Some sufferers will remain chronically ill, debilitated by the obsessional disorder, while others will achieve partial or complete recovery. The character traits that we see in persons suffering from obsessional disorders, like difficulty with flexibility, intimate relationships, and decision making, are issues that must be worked on throughout one's life.

The factor that most influences an individual's ability to overcome OCD is chronicity: How long has someone been afflicted with the disorder? How invested in the symptoms is he? How much of a sense of emptiness has he to overcome? What was the age at onset of the disorder? Many persons state that they began obsessive-compulsive behavior around the age of nine. If this is generally true for sufferers, then one needs to evaluate how much of the individual's adolescent development was impaired. Were peer relationships formed? Social groups joined? Was psychosexual development normal throughout the adolescent period (if the patient is an adult)?

What becomes obvious is that OCD assessment and prognosis is the same as for other psychological and psychiatric disorders. Other factors in forming a prognosis include the existence of secondary diagnoses. Does the individual suffer from other disabling disorders? Those that usually accompany OCD are depression and anxiety. When thought disorders (schizophrenia and/or psychosis) accompany OCD, there is another primary diagnosis made. (In such cases thought disorders would be the primary diagnosis.)

External and stress factors are the same for OCD sufferers (in their ability to facilitate or inhibit recovery) as for other psychological disorders. The presence of resourceful support persons like family or close friends can facilitate change. A gratifying job placement helps. The absence of these kinds of support factors tends to reinforce the individual's desire to remain emotionally separate from others and to continue to use self-soothing rituals to regulate anxiety and depression.

Assessment, then, includes the patient's current lifestyle. How completely organized around OCD rituals is it? If the patient is married, is the spouse an enabler, supporting the ritualized behaviors? If the patient is an adolescent, or younger, does the family condone the illness? Can members of the family become involved in treatment, assisting the patient in a reconnecting or bonding process with them? Are they willing to constructively interfere with the illness and tolerate the patient's heightened anxiety?

Most victims of OCD exempt themselves from following their special patterns when the situation (socially or professionally) makes them too awkward to pursue. These patterns are most intense and relentless at home, either with or without the family present. Assessment includes an evaluation of how conflict-avoidant and how invested in maintaining the emotional and behavioral status quo key members of the patient's family are. How much energy is available from family for changes in their pattern of acceptance of OCD?

If lack of attachment (to people) and physical isolation (severe needs for privacy) foster the opportunity for OCD rituals, then both areas must be modified simultaneously. Obviously this is easier to achieve with a child or adolescent living at home with his or her family, and the most difficult to achieve with an adult living alone. The therapist may initially have to be the sole resource person for the latter. In the case of children and adolescents, a therapist needs to work with parents to help them get closer to their child while constructively interfering with OCD rituals.

Olivia (whom we met on the very first page of this book) is a good example. At age fifteen, she came to her initial consultation session at her mother's request. According to her mother, she was engaged in so many OCD rituals that some days she did not attend school in order to complete her list from the previous day. Olivia was pleasant and engaging and indicated to me that she thought she did not need help and that she "had everything under control." She thanked me for my time, explaining that her mother was overconcerned and tended to exaggerate.

That evening I received a call from Olivia's mother, who asked me to phone her daughter and tell her to come in for a second meeting. I explained that this would be an ineffective approach and would put me in the position of pursuing Olivia and seeming like one more helpless person in her life. I told Mrs. B. that the alternate mode of treatment was to have her come in herself for regular therapy in order to make her the primary person who could create change in Olivia. Her initial reaction was that this sounded like an overwhelming role for her to play, that a person of her limited abilities did not know enough about psychology to do this. I assured her that what she did not know she could learn, and that we were more concerned with changing a pattern between herself and her daughter than with her acquiring a working knowledge of psychology.

In our first meeting we discussed Olivia's style of living at home. I asked, "What is it like for you to spend a day at home with Olivia?"

"There is no such thing as spending a day with Olivia. She may be at home, but it's hard to tell where she is, and often I will stay away from that part of the house because I'm afraid of what I will see. I really don't like to see her doing these strange rituals, touching parts of her body before getting dressed, twisting this way, then that way. It's gotten to the point where I can't tell if what she is doing at a particular time is a normal behavior or a ritual. Most of the time it seems like she is doing rituals. Then again, I think that I may have blown it all out of proportion . . . but not really."

"At this point, then, Olivia is free to perform her rituals, unhampered by you or your husband?"

"I hope that my husband doesn't notice, because sometimes he just screams at her that she's crazy. I'm sure that isn't good for her. Afterward he feels bad, so he stays away from her for days. I just don't say anything. I feel so sad for Olivia, but her need to do all the strange things she does—it seems so powerful."

"Does it feel like there's a lot of distance between you and your daughter?"

"She talks to me, but I feel like I don't know her anymore. If I ever question her about what she's doing, she has a temper tantrum. She gets so nasty, calls me stupid, shouts at me. Sometimes she seems like a monster. I don't want to do anything that will make her worse."

"Does the fear of making her worse affect the way you talk to her?"

She did not answer me directly. "My daughter's very strange," she said, "but she still makes sense when she talks. I mean, she's not crazy. What if I push her over the edge? She does crazy things, actions that aren't necessary or even sensible, but she talks like a sane person. Who knows, maybe she could get worse. And then she would really be a crazy person. I don't want that for her."

"So your fear of her getting worse gives her more privacy to do more rituals, which in effect makes her worse but not crazy."

She sighed and nodded her head in agreement. "So you see what I'm up against. No matter what I do, she gets worse."

I said, "It's clear that currently you can't help her. Does this also limit your ability to be comforting to her, to be warm and affectionate?"

"Affectionate? Forget about that! If I try to give her a hug, she shrugs away from me and suggests that my hands are sticky, or that in some way I will contaminate her. As for being warm or supportive, I just don't feel she wants anything from me anymore." Mrs. B. became tearful.

"Are there other members of your family who do want something from you?"

"My husband and my other daughter, Theresa—Terri, we call her—she is completely normal. She hugs, she kisses, she takes advice . . . sometimes she's fresh like all kids, but she knows how to ask for help. That's what surprised me about Olivia. She's the younger one. Terri was difficult as a kid, more argumentative. Olivia was a little angel. She slept the night, after four weeks, anyway. We didn't have any trouble until she was six. That year, my mother died and Olivia was afraid to be in a different room from me. We couldn't leave her with baby-sitters for a year after that, and she found it difficult to go to school. Then a cousin, my brother's daughter, died of leukemia two years later. It was terrible for all of us. Olivia became afraid of the dark. She was eight then. None of this affected Terri, who was eleven, strongly. It was about a year later that I first noticed Olivia was being fussy about the way she did things. She washed her hands a lot. She changed her clothes after school, and then again before dinner. I just thought it was a stage she'd outgrow."

"Did your husband notice this at the time?"

"My husband was doing a lot of traveling for his company, especially at that time. I'm not sure he was home enough to notice. When he was, he was usually exhausted. Things are better for him now. He doesn't travel quite as much."

"If your husband travels a lot, then you have to manage both girls. I guess you're used to being completely in charge of the house?"

"When my husband is home, he's in charge. He needs to feel he is, so I let him."

"What if you didn't make it look like he was in control?"

"I think he could adjust to it. He really knows he isn't."

"I will encourage you to act toward Olivia as if her secret wish was for you to take complete care of her, as if she were much younger than she is."

Mrs. B. began laughing. "It's one thing for you to tell me that I shouldn't continue to make it look as if my husband's in charge. We have a good marriage; he'll cooperate. But you're asking me to act as if my daughter wants me to be in charge of her." Again, she laughed. "If that's her secret, she's sure fooled me."

I asked Mrs. B. to bring Olivia in with her for an evaluation of the way they related to each other.

Several days later they entered the room together, with Mrs. B. following Olivia to the couch. When Olivia saw that her mother was going to sit next to her, she got up and sat in the armchair. Mrs. B. seemed embarrassed, Olivia looked annoyed. Arching her back, she sat very high in the chair; Mrs. B. slumped round-shouldered on the couch.

I began, "There seems to be a difference of opinion about whether Olivia's behavior needs to be viewed as a sign of difficulty or not. Olivia, in my first meeting with you, you indicated that you believed that your mother was making too much of the way you do things."

Olivia said, "I think she's just trying to embarrass me here."

"I'm not trying to embarrass you," said her mother quickly. "I'm trying to help you."

"I don't need that kind of help, thank you."

"Then . . . what do you need, honey?"

As the conversation between them continued, Mrs. B. appeared to be in retreat. Her voice rose as she reached the end of each sentence. As a result, all of her statements sounded like questions. Her daughter's posture began as assertive and shifted toward contemptuous.

I interjected, "Do you always take these roles in terms of each other?"

"What do you mean?" asked Olivia.

"When I listen to both of you, if I didn't pay attention to what you were discussing but only listened to your tone, I would hear you sounding annoyed, perhaps even fed up, with your mother. And you . . ." I turned to Mrs. B. ". . . sound like you are apologizing for bringing Olivia here, for inquiring about how she sees herself. In general, you seem apologetic toward her. I was wondering if it's always like this between you?"

Olivia said, "No, we usually get along fine. It's just when my mother harps on the same old things, I get frustrated." Suddenly she became tearful. Surprised at seeing her daughter so vulnerable, Mrs. B.'s eyes also welled up with tears, but she suppressed them at that point. I kept talking to Olivia so that she would not notice her mother's sadness.

During our next individual session, I asked Mrs. B., "What were you experiencing when Olivia was scolding you?"

"It just felt like the usual. She often talks to me like that. She knows it all. Sometimes she's like a brick wall."

"Did it feel the same when you were watching her talk to me?"

Again Mrs. B. became tearful, but this time as she talked she allowed herself to cry. "No. It felt different to watch her talk with you. Excuse me. I don't mean to get choked up. I just felt so sad for her. It was strange. I liked her better when she was talking to you."

"Why do you think you liked her better?"

"Well, I mean, it's not that I don't love Olivia. I always love her. It's just that she can be so difficult, so defensive, so obnoxious. I want to shake her and say, 'Stop this craziness!' Then I become afraid that I'll make her worse, so I don't say anything at all. When she was speaking to you she was more honest than she is with me. She *is* unhappy. She *is* frightened. She'll never show that to me. She'll just berate me, be patronizing. If I push her hard enough, she'll become shrill and hysterical, so I back off."

"What do you think it looks like to Olivia when you do that?"

Mrs. B. smiled in a self-mocking way. "Do you remember what you said to us when Olivia and I were here together? How I sound apologetic? Well, I'm sure that's true. The instant she becomes shrill, I'm sure my eyebrows go up, my voice gets shaky and sorry in tone, and then she becomes angry, almost nasty, but calmer. And she usually stalks off and slams a door or two."

"I guess this is a regular pattern between you?"

"Well, frankly, I try to avoid the angry-hysterical part as much as I can. I just walk on eggshells around her most of the time."

"You said that you liked her more when she was talking to me. Does that mean she's not so likable to you when you're walking on eggshells?"

"No. I guess I don't feel so good about her when it's like that."

"Why do you think Olivia became vulnerable with me?"

"I'm not sure. You were more comfortable asking her confrontational questions than I am."

"Maybe I have more faith in her sanity than you do. You said that you were afraid your anger might make her worse. Confrontation and anger don't have to be the same thing."

She looked puzzled for a moment. "I don't think I ever thought of that. If I could confront her without being afraid of or angry at her, she would be more vulnerable. But she wouldn't, not with me. Maybe our relationship is just too thoroughly formed."

"So you have the same pessimism about change that your daughter has. If you can't do it immediately, then you can never do it."

"Do you really think our pattern, which is God knows how old, can be changed?"

"I think that a fifteen-year-old girl is still open to parenting from her mother."

She looked at me challengingly. "So what's the first change I should make?"

"Your voice should not rise in inflection at the end of your sentences. They all sound like questions, even when they aren't. You sound stronger if your voice remains even. Olivia will hear that the first time you try it, and she will try to test your resolve."

"Won't this produce trouble at home? Won't things get noisier?"

"Yes. It will be part of her resistance to change. You'll have to tolerate that."

"But will my husband? When he comes home from work he wants quiet."

I shook my head. "He can have quiet and a sick daughter or noise and a recovering daughter. The bellowing, hopefully, will be made by your daughter and not by you or your husband."

Mrs. B. agreed. She had needed an ally, for she did not have sufficient confidence in herself. This was one of the things her daughter was angry about. Now Mrs. B. could gain confidence by utilizing the therapist for the emotional support she needed to parent her daughter.

The prognosis for Olivia in individual psychotherapy would have been poor. She did not want to be in therapy, and she thought that nothing was wrong. The outlook changed markedly for the better when her mother proved to be resourceful and willing to change her usual ways of coping with Olivia's illness. They had a more confrontational and very loud relationship for several months, which then tapered off to brief, infrequent episodes.

Over the course of two years, Olivia gave up most of her rituals and became positively attached to her mother. She had worked through enough dependency needs with her now more powerful and attractive mother and was ready to go to a residential college.

Mrs. B. had needed encouragement to see herself as the

important person she was to her daughter. She felt affection for her daughter, but Olivia discouraged the timid offers, and Mrs. B. became demoralized by Olivia's rejection of her care. She felt that she presented her loving feelings in an inadequate way and tried to project even more tenderness toward her daughter. But Olivia saw this increase of tenderness as an indication of weakness on the part of her mother.

Although Mrs. B. was nurturing, she was not authoritative enough to be respected by her daughter. While Mrs. B. was intimidated by her daughter's contemptuousness, Olivia had a secret wish for her mother to be more powerful. Mrs. B., in turn, needed a support person to advise her and empower her to be assertive with her daughter. After all, Mrs. B. was a competent woman who coped well with her life, in general, and her daughter had reached a point where she was not competent to cope with the demands of her life.

Once Mrs. B. was able to accept her sadness about her daughter and Olivia's lack of competence, she was able to restructure their relationship. While Olivia did not make it easy for her mother—she fought every change—she was secretly wishing for her mother to overpower her. As their relationship changed over the next two years, Olivia gradually became more attracted to her mother and less driven to her rituals. As Olivia became more compliant with her mother's wishes for her to reduce her dependency on rituals, Olivia's mother felt a growing sense of competence and increased her authoritative requests for her daughter to change. The cycle reinforced itself with increasing momentum. Olivia became rebonded with her mother in a therapeutic return to a more childlike relationship.

Ultimately, Olivia would have to do some separating from her mother to achieve her own adulthood, a process that could take another five years. But many victims of OCD, if untreated, suffer limitations throughout their lifetimes. Although treatment may include years of psychotherapy, reparenting, and, sometimes, medication, this is surely preferable to a lifetime disability.

THIRTEEN

Turning Points

There are two kinds of turning points in the treatment of OCD. The first is the development of some optimism about the availability of a trustworthy, dependable person, either the psychotherapist or the parent in charge (such as Olivia's mother, who actively worked on the problems of a child suffering from OCD). The second turning point is the lessening of the patient's stress, the anxiety or anxious depression that the patient is suffering from. For symptoms to begin to abate, both kinds of turning points will need to occur.

The first turning point is reached through a successful connection, bonding, or engagement in treatment with a therapist. This can also be a rebonding with a parent who has worked hard to intensify the connection she or he has with the child or adolescent sufferer. The point at which the patient is able to feel reassurable by the therapist or parent is the beginning of therapeutic change.

The second turning point is achieved by changes in the patient's life: family relationships, school, work, sense of achievement, or self-esteem. Sometimes a patient can utilize therapy to become the initiator of the change. This can be done by the patient's deliberate reduction of time spent alone doing rituals. This is followed by a self-conscious period of outgoing behavior on the part of the patient until comfort with the new behavior is achieved.

Sometimes, no matter how solid the therapeutic connection, the patient's level of anxiety or agitated depression does not allow her to risk new behaviors or give up any rituals. It is at that point that medication needs to be considered to permit the patient to get to the second point. With medication reducing the emotional factors that perpetuate the use of rituals, and a strong connection to the therapist who relieves the patient's despair about dependency, symptoms should begin to subside.

A patient once asked me, "What do you mean when you say I need to learn to be dependent?"

I answered with a question. "What does 'depend' mean?" But before she could answer, I went to the bookshelf in my office and brought out *Webster's New World Dictionary.* "Here," I said, handing her the book. "Find the word *depend* and read what it says."

She did, turning quickly to the word and reading aloud. "It means 'To be influenced or determined by something else. To be contingent on. To have trust; rely on. To rely on for support or aid.'"

Nodding, I told her, "Now think what that means concerning yourself. You aren't able to do any of that. You can't be influenced or determined by anything or anybody outside yourself. You can't bring yourself to trust anyone for support or aid. You can't rely on anyone or be contingent on anyone. And that's why you have to go right on coping with your anxiety by using those rituals—unless you can learn how to depend on someone."

In the cases of Lara and Olivia, they learned to depend on their mothers. The turning points for both of them were when they recognized their mothers' assertiveness toward them, and understood that they would be protected by their parents' stronger postures. For differing periods of time (months for Lara and weeks for Olivia) both girls sulked and had tantrums in resistance to change. Their outbursts represented their conflict that their mothers would not be able to make them feel as secure as the rituals did. But their mothers' caring firmness won them over, and they gave up their rituals. This intensive involvement was required for several years afterward to solidify the girls' new style of seeking security.

The turning point for Lauren was surprising. She was, you will recall, both psychiatrist and patient and had great difficulty accepting the posture of a patient. I anticipated that much time would be required before this would diminish sufficiently to make successful treatment possible, but such was not the case. The turning point came when Lauren tried to kill herself. But it was not a true attempt, for although she swallowed a lethal dose of prescription medication plus alcohol, she made phone calls to ensure that she would fail. But her actions made it necessary for her to be placed in the hospital overnight, and this is what produced the turning point.

Lauren experienced the medical care in the hospital as extremely humiliating, for it made her (the psychiatrist) feel far more mentally ill than she normally regarded herself. The shock of this humiliation had two results: First, it discouraged any future suicide attempts, real or unreal. Second, it caused Lauren, with the therapist's help, to begin working away from seeing herself as the sick and crazy person she had lived with so long.

Although there would be a long period during which she tested me as her therapist to see if I would be overwhelmed by her, to see if I would discharge or dismiss her, she was on her way toward giving up all her self-harming behavior and to realizing she was not too much for me to cope with.

In the case of Claudia, the daughter of an alcoholic father whom we met in chapter 4, the turning point came when she, like Lauren, resorted to self-mutilation and I as her therapist did not reenact her parents' response to her. (They had placed her in a psychiatric hospital for a year when she was thirteen.) Her mother's comment at the time was, "What have I done that you should end up like this?" Her father's comment was, "This is the stupidest thing you've ever done."

My comment upon being told by Claudia that she had cut herself was, "Let me see your arm."

"I don't like showing you this," she told me, pulling her arm away as soon as I had seen it.

"It doesn't look like it needs a physician's attention. Have you had a tentanus shot recently?"

Looking sullen, she was waiting for me to become overwhelmed by her act and abandon her as being beyond my ability to help (just as her parents had done). I dealt with the cut as a first-aid issue and an enactment of her need to present me with her most difficult-to-nurture self, in effect, to test me before risking placing her trust in me. This was the hidden Claudia, very different from the flip, glib Claudia who competed with me for dominance in earlier sessions.

At one point in that session, Claudia asked me, "Don't you think that I should be put away [in a psychiatric hospital]?"

"No, but I do think if you stay this overwhelmed we should see about medication for you. That's the next step."

She was surprised at the mildness of my response. "You don't think that I'm too much for you?"

"No. I think you've come to the right place."

I did tell Claudia that I did not want her to cut herself anymore. If she felt upset, she was supposed to call me; she was able to use my not wanting her to hurt herself as a reason not to. Within months, she was also able to use this rationale to give up alcohol. So intense was her well-disguised need to connect with someone that within a year much of her compulsive exercising had abated.

Turning points with compulsive cleanliness tend to show more gradual improvement. In the cases of Alice (chapter 5) and Ashley (chapter 1 and chapter 8), the turning points for them were less concise. It was a matter of my being consistent in posture over a long period of time in my role as therapist. The success of the attachment process was demonstrated by the patient's willingness to ask me for advice. Then I became a counselor, and in so doing was able to give the patient advice. The dialogue established around advice giving can be much like a parent's relationship with a son or daughter. If the advice fails, the therapist is held responsible within the relationship. Arguing may even develop. This is healthy, providing it is done responsibly, and it can further deepen trust. When advisory issues come up with regard to the necessity of cleanliness rituals, then a turning point is reached. When a patient asks if a particular ritual is really necessary, this tells us how secure the patient feels with the therapist. But it will still be some time before rituals subside.

Diane (whom we met in chapter 4 and who will be discussed more fully in the next chapter) experienced a turning point over the issue of boundaries. Without an invitation, she came to my table in a coffee shop and sat down. When I suggested that we not begin our session there but wait until we were upstairs in the office, she dismissed my objection, advising me that, "You could just pretend I'm not here."

I postponed my reply for ten minutes. When we arrived upstairs, I was angry with her but wanted to do something constructive with it. We entered the office knowing that we were about to have an argument. I began, "I want to talk to you about boundaries. When I'm in the coffee shop, I am not your therapist."

"That's okay. I didn't expect you to be my therapist in the coffee shop."

I responded, "My understanding is that whenever we are together for more than a brief encounter, I am your therapist."

"I don't agree with you. I know you eat breakfast at that coffee shop, and I like it, too. So why can't I eat breakfast there?"

"But you didn't eat breakfast there before you had appointments with me at eight in the morning."

"Well, now it's convenient for me to eat there."

"I feel it's an invasion of my privacy when you schedule

yourself into my breakfast. To protect that privacy, I will have to change your appointment to later in the day."

She paused, then said a surprising thing, "I don't know why, but that makes me feel safer. I mean your threat to change my appointment makes me feel better, and that's weird."

"I didn't make the threat in order to make you feel safe, just to protect my privacy. But I'm curious about your response. Why do you think it makes you feel safer?"

"I guess that I believe I mess up a lot of relationships, and this could be one of them. I guess I like the idea that you are stopping me from screwing this one up, too."

One of Diane's rituals was to spend hours in Manhattan coffee shops watching the customers from the safety of her crossword puzzle book. When she wanted to expand that ritual to include watching me, I had unwittingly taken control of what, emotionally, she regarded as her territory: the coffee shop. She experienced my reaction as constructive interference. Over the next two years most of the time she had spent on rituals was gradually returned to the social sphere. She enrolled in graduate school and began dating for the first time.

Another sign that a turning point has been reached is when a patient becomes more impatient and resentful about feeling compelled to perform rituals to regulate anxiety. Initially, there exists a greater alliance between the patient and her rituals than there is between patient and therapist. As treatment progresses, it clearly evolves into an alliance of patient and therapist against the compulsion to do those rituals.

Here is how one patient described the phenomenon of reaching one particular type of turning point, that moment when a ritual is dropped from its usual place, time, or circumstance: "I just stopped taking extra showers. It felt weird. I felt like something was missing . . . unfamiliar. I reminded myself that it was good that I skipped the showers. It made me feel nervous and empty. I didn't like it. I hope these feelings go away."

The pattern of relinquishing rituals can be uneven, with

many relapses. A more gradual pattern of decreasing rituals was experienced by someone we've already met, Nina. She had left the hospital after regaining the weight she had lost due to her severely compulsive-ridden anorexia nervosa.

"When I first left the hospital, I had to eat dinner on six plates," she told me. "It drove the family crazy. One day my mother came in with two divider dinner plates. Each was split into three compartments. That was an easier change to adjust to. After six months, I cut down to one divider plate. I pretended that it was divided into six parts. It looked almost normal to my family. I guess I had to humor myself to get less compulsive. When I'm nervous, I still can pretend that a regular plate is divided into six parts. I move my food around discreetly, as if there were dividers separating it. Now I only do it when I'm really nervous, so I guess that's not so bad. Maybe someday I won't do it at all."

Turning points toward recovery vary in duration and intensity as much as the reasons for the onset of obsessive-compulsive disorders. In a previous chapter, we saw how some individuals were literally traumatized into their inward-turning rituals while others began doing ritualistic behavior for more subtle reasons. In the same way, someone occasionally reduces their ritualistic behavior dramatically after entering therapy. But this is unusual. More often, there is a gradual lessening of the rituals. Usually, one who has placed less intensity upon doing them "forgets" to do some of them part of the time. This "forgetting" continues until there is an observable decrease in the pattern.

For some the extinction of all ritual patterns occurs; for others some habits remain but are experienced as nuisances rather than life limiting. When psychotherapy and changes in relationships as well as environment don't produce significant improvements, additional treatment needs to be added to promote turning points.

FOURTEEN
Medication

Patients will sometimes say to me, "I see a lot of change in myself, but I don't know whether it's the therapy or the medication." This is certainly a question that psychotherapists ask themselves. Psychopharmacologists (psychiatrists who specialize in the prescribing of psychoactive medication) often attribute all disorders to constitutional problems and expect medication to resolve emotional problems that are diagnosed as psychiatric disorders. On the other hand, psychoanalytically trained psychotherapists often take the viewpoint that all of these emotional problems can be analyzed out of existence, and that the use of medication is simply a failure to work through conflicts analytically and, therefore, a false solution. Both groups, the psychopharmacologists and the psychoanalysts, often suffer from tunnel vision, each selectively ignorant of factors the other takes into consideration.

When medication is successful, it implies that an individual has been suffering from a constitutional disability—a mood or anxiety disorder that is biomedical in nature. This constitutional disability has made the individual more sensitive and vulnerable to family turmoil and life's difficulties than a constitutionally less vulnerable person would be. While no medication should be touted as the cure, some degree of success for a percentage of sufferers is clearly noted.

Consider the case of Diane and antidepressants. Diane, introduced in chapter 4, entered treatment one year after college graduation. She had remained at home, not attempting to find work or further education. Her days were ritual ridden. She spent at least two hours a day in Manhattan coffee shops, where, as previously mentioned, she would do crossword puzzles while watching and listening to diners. This was the social part of her day. During a year, partly as a result of her rigid eating patterns, she had developed atypical anorexia nervosa (she was not consciously concerned with losing weight as much as she was in not varying her inadequate eating patterns).

Diane was an outgoing personality until the age of sixteen when, as a passenger on the back of a motorbike, she and her companion were hit by a car. As a result she was in a coma for nine days. When she regained consciousness, it was apparent she had suffered substantial neurological impairment and had to learn to read and write again. She had lost her ability to do even simple arithmetic. (Her parents were resourceful, and tutored her on a daily basis.) In addition, her left shoulder and arm were shattered, and her left breast scarred. She and her family were told that even if the arm could be saved, she would probably not be able to use it, despite numerous operations over a five-year period. She regained her mental abilities and, due to her determination and tolerance for the most rigorous physiotherapy, regained the use of a weakened arm.

She completed high school and went off to college, determined to achieve in a manner that characterized her recovery. During her third year in college, she began to withdraw from other students. She lost weight and her routines became rigidified. Drifting away from her few remaining friends, she continued to succeed academically while developing a reclusive style during nonclass hours. After graduation, her rigid pattern with its isolation and rituals continued and deepened.

During her initial interview with me, she presented her medical history with a grandiose flamboyance. She was proud of what she had achieved in terms of her medical recovery. "They said that I would never be able to use my arm again," she told me. And she unbuttoned her blouse and rolled up her sleeve, exposing the left half of her upper body. "It's been through hell, and so have I."

Her breast was severely scarred, the muscle configurations in the arm partially distorted. Some of the white lines of scar tissue indicated the impact of the accident on her arm and shoulder; others were the signature of surgical reconstructions. She extended the arm in my direction, not so much for me to inspect it, but more to confront me with her disfigurement.

"You have no idea how many operations I've had on this," she told me, nodding at the arm, which she was still extending, supporting it with her right hand. "And the physiotherapy was excruciating. I must have screamed in the physiotherapist's ear dozens of times . . . But now I can use it." Her style was different from most victims of OCD, as well as most anorexics. She was outgoing, highly disclosing, and assertive on the first meeting.

My response was, "I can see that you've been through an enormous ordeal."

She shrugged, rebuttoning her blouse. "Not really. It's over now, anyway."

"And you're not here because of your arm, are you?"

"No. I'm here because I'm weird."

"What kind of weird are you?"

"My parents can't stand the way I do things. They hound me every day about everything."

"What does everything include?"

"It includes the time I wake up in the morning, and all my routines: my shopping trips, my crossword puzzles, eating in bed, the way I wear my hair, the times of the day that I do things, how often I go to the bathroom. You name it, and they don't like it."

"Do *you* like them—all the things they complain about?"

"It depends. Some I like, and some I don't."

"Well then, what is it that I can do for you?"

"That's a good question. I'm not sure of the answer." Her response was playful and elusive, perhaps defiant.

"I'm clearer on what I can do for your parents," I told her.

"What do you mean?"

"I'm sure they have definite ideas about your getting rid of your weirdness."

She smiled mischievously. "I'm sure they would agree with you about that."

"You have me dazzled with your heroism regarding your arm, a story you can tell comfortably and have probably told before; but as near as I can see, you're almost completely inaccessible."

"What do you mean?" she asked, grabbing her left shoulder.

I paused, touched by her relationship with her arm. "I guess after all these years of a lack of physical privacy, you have learned to uncover yourself and put yourself on physical display for doctors, nurses, and physiotherapists. Perhaps because you've had to relinquish physical separateness, you have to withdraw into inaccessibility emotionally, even while appearing so outgoing."

She stared blankly at me. After a minute or so, her eyes welled up. As the tears streamed down her cheeks, she turned her face toward the ceiling, trying to hide them in this unusual manner.

I said, "Maybe I could help you develop some physical modesty . . . while you learn to expose your feelings."

Now she began to cry aloud. "But I have no life," she sobbed. "Everything that I do my parents hate, and they're probably right. What if I can never have a life? What if I can never stop doing all these things?"

The things that Diane was engaged in doing, and her drive to do them, were intense. This included OCD rituals, anorexic weight-controlling behavior, and rigorous exercise. And, in contrast to her abstaining from eating throughout the day, she would binge in bulimic style until two in the morning on low-calorie foods.

Depressed in reaction to the empty life she had been leading for three years, she was in distress due to the aftermath of her accident; no matter how hard she struggled (and she was used to excelling), her arm would never look or function normally. In addition, she may have been experiencing posttrauma induced by depression. In family consultation sessions, both Diane and her parents expressed the belief that her personality had changed after the accident, and the contrast remained.

Diane's weight was twenty pounds below normal. We agreed that when she gained ten pounds, I would send her for a psychopharmacological consultation since her weight was below the range where it is believed that antidepressants are effective. After four months in treatment, Diane reached ninety pounds, her short-term goal. She was placed on an antidepressant that helped her relinquish much of her obsessive-compulsive behavior. This was of great importance. In addition, Diane worked hard to reduce the frequency of each behavior and to eliminate others. The most stubborn behaviors proved to be her eating rituals, even though she was in the process of normalizing her weight.

One day she came in with the following complaint: "This antidepressant is helping me with some of my rituals, but it does nothing for my eating or my depression."

With my encouragement and with help from the psychopharmacologist, Diane discontinued this medication and began a second antidepressant, one that did help with her eating and her depression as well. She never resumed her OCD behaviors. After a year on this medication, she enrolled in graduate school, and after four more months tapered her second medication to what would be termed a subclinical dosage. At this point, she experienced no depression, and she considered herself an eccentric eater, though she would not fulfill the diagnostic criteria for an eating disorder.

Diane's therapy sessions had taken place twice each week while she struggled with issues of separation from her parents.

She described herself as having been independent from her parents before the accident, but physically and psychologically thrown back to an infantile situation with them during her convalescence. Her parents had been relentlessly noncompliant with all of her OCD and eating-disordered behavior. They continued that posture during her first year of therapy. When they saw positive changes in her weight and some lessening of ritualistic behavior, they became less engaged in protesting her activities. For Diane, the prolonging of a childish relationship with her parents created personality problems that had to be worked out in therapy.

"I've always liked the spotlight," she told me. "You know, before my accident, I was a dancer. I was popular, with lots of friends. After the accident, I was the center of attention for my parents and the doctors. As soon as I could, I took on a peformance role with them. I kept reassuring them that I would make a quick recovery, the quickest ever seen. I knew that I looked terrible, that my arm looked terrible, that the whole situation looked terrible. I felt like I was carrying the ball, keeping everyone's morale up. That way I was the perfect patient. I was special; I was the star."

"What's so important about being a star?"

"I don't know. I guess it feels better than *not* being the star."

"How long has it been since you've felt connected to anyone in a personal way, since anyone has gotten to know you very well?"

Her answer had a manicky lilt to it. "Oh who can tell? Maybe eight or nine years."

"Is being a star 'justified isolation'?"

"What do you mean?"

"Well, a star is separate from the audience, and even the other performers. I was wondering if separateness is at the center of your idea of being a star."

"I don't know. My parents are always complaining about my separateness. They're always on my case about being alone, especially the time I spend in coffee shops." She paused, then resumed her manicky tone. "It's wonderful to be a star, to be special. I've always wanted to excel. I don't want to be ordinary or treated like an average person. I like doing my crossword puzzles. It's fun to watch people in the coffee shops. Sometimes I do it for hours. I get a corner table where I can see everybody, and sometimes I talk to people; other times I just watch them. Do you think I should give it all up? I don't think so."

"I felt like you were just having a conversation with yourself."

"What's wrong with that?"

"If you're with other people and you go on as if they weren't there, then you're vulnerable to not knowing what their reaction to you is. You lose track of them, perhaps fearing their disapproval, but it's not protection because you may pay social penalties for your lack of awareness of others' needs . . . Maybe the real trouble is you're afraid that you don't fit in."

Her stare became focused again. "So you disapprove?"

"Let's just say I would find it boring being lectured at if we were having a social conversation and you took that tone with me. If you want to be the star and you want me to play the audience, it won't work. It probably won't work with anyone."

She became somber and reflective. She put her chin in the palm of her hand, her elbow resting on her right knee. "So maybe that's why I prefer to be alone. Maybe I'm just no good at being with people. Maybe I never will be, and this is my compensation."

"I guess that the same way you had to learn reading and arithmetic all over again, you can redevelop your social skills to whatever they need to become."

She looked up at me, chin in hand, eyebrows raised. "Do you have any idea how much I need to develop to become normal?"

"Are you overwhelmed by the prospect?"

"I'm scared to death by the prospect. You mentioned me being so comfortable uncovering my body for people to inspect after my accident. Well, obviously there are areas that I'm not so comfortable with. I'm a twenty-three-year-old virgin, and I'm afraid I'll wind up a forty-six-year-old virgin, and maybe a ninety-two-year-old virgin."

"You said that with bravado, much the same bravado with which you uncovered your arm."

"What's the difference how I said it? I'm scared of sex! Okay?"

"The difference is that you have a lot of difficulty communicating in a straightforward manner, and I'm going to call your attention to the way you communicate—your style, tone, and everything else that enables you to distance yourself from the person you're talking to."

"But I may need the distance," she protested.

"Tell me about the physical therapy after surgery."

"I don't see what that has to do with anything . . . but okay. By the way, have you ever had physiotherapy?"

"No."

"Well, it's not exactly thrilling. Well, in sort of a cockeyed way, I guess it is. You get to see how much pain you can endure. You get into a contest with yourself. After my surgery, my elbow was so stiff it felt like I didn't have a joint there at all. Then I would be visited by this guy. He was very big and very strong, and he would take my arm and bend it until I would scream . . . and I always held out as long as I could. No matter how long I held out, he would bend until I screamed."

"That sounds frightening and painful."

"You can bet your life on it."

"Did you get mad at the physiotherapist?"

"Sure. I cursed at him plenty."

"So I guess you'll get mad at me, too."

"If you're going to put me through that kind of shit, yeah, I'll get mad at you."

"Putting up with that pain is why you beat the odds and can use your arm."

She nodded vigorously.

"And so," I said, "when you communicate in an offputting style, I may have to bend it with confrontation."

She smiled. "I guess all therapy is one kind of pain or another."

Not long after that conversation, Diane began to date a man.

In the past, she had not dated anyone more than twice. If by that time she had not discouraged him with her refusal to eat a meal with him or display even the most casual affection, she would outright refuse to date him a third time.

"I never feel any connection with anyone I date," she had told me. "If they looked good from a distance, by the time I've gone out with them once, I've lost all interest. I feel that it's misleading to go out with them again. Besides, they might expect something in the way of romance from me. I haven't got those feelings for anybody I've dated, so why bother?"

Diane's characterization of her feelings toward dating changed when she came in and announced, "I'm dating this fellow for the fourth time, and I'm still interested in him."

"I guess you feel safer about getting close to him than you have with other men."

She looked at me mischievously. "Not just safer—interested, excited . . ." Her enthusiasm dwindled. ". . . and ignorant. I don't know what I'm supposed to do. I don't know how I'm supposed to behave . . . sexually."

"What do you think he expects of you?"

"Probably that I should know what I'm doing . . . Look, I don't know how to say this, but I'm afraid of . . . penises. I don't think that they're attractive, and I don't want to have much to do with them . . . I mean, what is expected of me?"

"You aren't expected to do anything you don't want to do."

"But don't guys expect all kinds of service?"

"You think that you should seem expert at this?"

"Well, everybody talks a good game."

"Perhaps this is a good way for you to be the receiver of care rather than the provider. I guess one of the scariest aspects of this for you is that you can't be in control, the giver of care, the expert. And on top of it all, you're scared. Why don't you be *his* problem? Why not let your ignorance and your preferences be something *he* must contend with?"

"That's scarier than the sex."

"*Or* that's why the sexual part seems scary."

"So I don't have to worry about it?"

"No. You'll probably have to be honest about your experience . . . or lack of it."

"That won't turn him off?"

"If it does, you'll just have to write him off as a loss."

"But I don't have to fake anything?"

"If you do, then you'll have fake sex."

"That doesn't sound so good."

For a variety of reasons, conducting psychotherapy with people suffering with obsessional disorders involves teaching, counseling, and advising, and this may include talking about sexual matters. Many OCD patients lack experience in this area due to their propensity for social isolation.

For Diane to have asked me the questions she did meant that she had developed a level of trust that enabled her to transcend her previous obsessional isolation. To ask her to analyze her feelings about sexuality at that point would be to abandon her. To offer advice, which she could accept or reject, was her interpersonal request. The nature of therapy for her at this point (the first two years) was to use the material she presented to enhance an interpersonal dialogue, to assist her to make a connection, and to increase that connection within appropriate boundaries.

Diane presented the kinds of interpersonal problems that required more confrontations, initially, than support. These difficulties kept her isolated socially, which reinforced her reclusive behavior and her OCD rituals, along with other rigid behavior patterns. They were not OCD specifically, but served the same purpose—the regulation of mood and anxiety without the assistance of others. They maintained her isolation and fears of being socially inadequate, which by this time she had become. In effect, part of her therapy had to become a sort of sheltered workshop in social interaction. The here and now between Diane and the therapist had to be analyzed and often confronted, not as transference, but as a struggle between two people. Diane was able to put this "painful therapy" in perspective and value it as challenging honesty. She was also able to understand that confrontation was not persecution and did not mean that she was disliked.

The therapeutic dynamic that interfered with her OCD was her attraction to the frank confrontation (on her behalf) that was taking place between herself and the therapist. This therapeutic connection allowed her to struggle with her core problem of isolation, to stay connected to that other person, and to use that relationship to regulate her moods and anxiety.

This is not to underestimate the value of her parents' behavior, which she found bothersome. They refused to disenfranchise themselves as social resources and agents of change. They were stubborn in their constructive demand for her normalcy, despite their own painful feelings about the extensive suffering caused by the accident.

The importance of medication for Diane must not be underestimated. Planned as short-term, it proved to be necessary for the indefinite future. After two years, still feeling guilty about using medication, Diane attempted to discontinue it. In consultation with a psychopharmacologist, she tapered her dosage in order to avoid withdrawal symptoms that might be confused with her normal, nonmedicated state.

After a period of six weeks off medication, Diane told me in a session, "I just feel pessimistic about everything, but nothing is going wrong. As a matter of fact, lots of things are going right. But somehow that doesn't help. I can see that I'm drifting back toward some of my old isolated behaviors again."

I asked, "Does this feeling, and your drifting back, have anything to do with the period of time that you have discontinued medication?"

She looked forlorn, raised her eyebrows and nodded in reluctant agreement. "Yeah. I think I'll have to resume medication again. I don't like the idea, but it works."

* * *

A major part of my responsibility as Diane's therapist was to help her learn to live with her medication without a sense of guilt or depression.

When medication is effective, it can produce dramatic reductions in ritualistic behavior within two weeks; and when coupled with effective psychotherapy, this reduction can become permanent.

FIFTEEN

The Medication Dilemma

Each of us is born with differing emotional sensitivities. Some children are clearly tenser or moodier than others. Some develop feeding problems in infancy or sleep disorders in early childhood. Are these differences the result of the infant's keen sensitivity to what's wrong with a mother, father, or the family system? Are there constitutional factors at work: digestive, muscular, neurological, even cognitive? Or are both present?

There are some who believe a single stress-oriented chemical change is responsible for the difference. Recently an experienced psychiatrist, who limits his practice to psychopharmacology, commented to me, "Steve, our group feels that many of the patients we see suffer from a broad-spectrum affective disorder, and we're not even sure whether the entities we call anxiety and depression are worth differentiating. There are simply these same chemical causes, but they produce different disorders in different people—depression or anxiety or obsessive-compulsive disorders. All from the same chemical cause."

The implications of this idea need clarification. If it is true, do all individuals develop this chemistry at the same age or stage of development? Can this chemical change be induced by trauma? By physical illness? If it is stress-oriented, does the chemical change cause the stress, or does the stress cause the chemical change? And if all disorders result from this chemical change, what dictates the particular form the change produces, be it anxiety, depression, phobias, obsessive-compulsive disorders, or alcoholism?

Even if we grant that a chemical change is the original culprit, this does not mean that it is solely responsible for the problem. Health-care specialists are not called in at the point where the original stress and chemical change occur. In the typical case, outward symptoms have reached the critical stage before help is sought. Where an individual, in reaction to family stress and constitutional vulnerability, has developed the coping behavior in OCD, much more than medication is required. The feelings of emptiness, lack of a sense of identity, difficulty with intimacy, attachment, and in being emotionally inaccessible to others—these results of the earlier interplay between constitutional vulnerability and family dysfunction can only be treated with psychotherapy.

Recently I was sharing a lecture program with a physician who was treating eating disorders using antidepressants. He described remarkable short-term results with some of his patients. But after he described their improvement, he shook his head and told the audience that he was discouraged and puzzled that those patients who achieved the *most* benefit from the medication usually discontinued the prescriptions and dropped out of treatment. And many of them, he subsequently discovered, relapsed.

During the question and answer period, I suggested to the physician that he did not have any business treating eating-disordered people without the collaboration of a psychotherapist, no more than I would agree to treat them without the collaboration of a physician. In the case of this doctor, his patients had no emotional support for living without their eating-disorder symptoms. Their feelings of emptiness, as well as their disappointment that life was not much improved with the loss of their symptoms, caused them to reenlist their eating-disordered behavior. In his single-faceted approach, he did not appreciate all the needs that symptoms signify for chronic sufferers. Nor did he understand the increasing emptiness that chronic use of symptomatic resolution alone both creates and fills.

Even to the extent that medication is successful, there are often psychological problems like guilt and depression associated with drug taking, as in the case of Diane. The question arises: Will it ever be possible to alter body chemistry with nonchemical means? The data required for a proper answer to this question may be years away, but currently available techniques as diverse as biofeedback, hypnosis, and medication offer hope for those who have the emotional resources to utilize such methods. Unfortunately, individuals who suffer from obsessive-compulsive disorders have little success with these disciplines, either because the patient's chemical disorder is too severe or because her defenses (rituals) are too well entrenched and too mind involving (obsessional).

For now, the best course of treatment utilizes psychotherapy and often, but not always, medication. It is unfortunate that within the mental health field there is often a lack of collaboration between medical and nonmedical psychodynamic psychotherapists, each competing in areas of diagnosis and mode of treatment, in some cases each seeing the other's point of view as threatening. There are innumerable case histories proving the benefit of teamwork. Remember Annabelle, in chapter 4?

Diagnostically, Annabelle suffered from obsessive-compulsive disorder, anorexia nervosa, bulimia, and a generalized anxiety disorder. She presented herself in a straightforward manner, requesting help in all areas. She proceeded to come to therapy sessions three times a week. Despite her long trip she rarely missed a session and was never late.

During the first several months of therapy, she recalled a history of obsessive-compulsive symptoms that reached back into childhood. She viewed her mother as a Jekyll and Hyde personality who could be the warmest, most caring, or the coldest, most distant person anyone would ever meet.

Annabelle explained that she lived in fear of her mother freezing her out. "She wouldn't talk to me for days at a time. I would apologize repeatedly . . . for anything and everything. I would never know exactly why the freeze-out would end, but as soon as it did, I anticipated the next one with dread."

She talked about her mother's need for closeness to her. "If I said I had a headache or anything that hurt me, my mother would suggest that I stay home from school with her for the day. It always seemed to me that she was happier when I was there."

She talked about her father's warmth, and his helplessness. "My father has told me recently that he used to feel so badly when my mother was cold to me that he would go into the other room and cry."

She described her mother's rigidity. "My mother must do the same thing every day. She gets up at the same time, makes each meal at a certain hour, does her exercises at a specific time of day, and then does her race-walking, timing it and counting her steps, not acknowledging neighbors in her path. She gets furious at anything that interferes with her schedule."

We can see reasons for anxiety existing in a child who constantly feared the next freeze-out from her mother, as well as feeling that her father was too insubstantial to depend upon at those times when her mother was emotionally inaccessible. It seems an adaptive compensation on Annabelle's part to utilize obsessive-compulsive rituals, since this kind of repetitious behavior calmed her anxiety without anyone else's assistance.

As her illness became more chronic, other features emerged. She became nearly housebound, her lifestyle resembling agoraphobia (the fear of leaving home), and she became fearful of neighbors observing her in the street near her house, of the checkers at the supermarket, and of other shopkeepers. She was experiencing some paranoia in this respect; Annabelle was a person whose existence had deteriorated to a never-ending series of rituals. Her own awareness of this motivated her cooperation in an intensive and multifaceted treatment.

Chronicity for someone with an obsessive-compulsive personality often means increased isolation from family and social relationships. It also produces a deepening of the behaviors and a proliferation of them until most thought processes and behaviors serve and follow obsessional patterns. It is no wonder that those chronically afflicted experience themselves as empty. Their obsessional constriction has confined them to a narrow mental frame devoid of intimacy and aesthetics.

While developmental causes abound for Annabelle's behavior, we cannot overlook the similarities between her symptoms and those of her mother. It is possible that her mother role-modeled obsessive-compulsive behavior for her daughter. Or perhaps there is a genetic transmission here. Does Annabelle's mother also experience the generalized anxiety disorder that Annabelle suffers from? There is much data missing. Both the current limitations of genetic research as well as the family's limitation on providing information offer a cluster of disorders whose origins we can only speculate on. In the face of such limitations, a therapeutic treatment and umbrella management approach that covers all possibilities must be constructed.

Due to her severe agitation, Annabelle was referred to a psychopharmacologist who prescribed a benzodiazepine for anxiety, and an antidepressant with obsessive-compulsive reduction properties. Here it was vitally important for the psychopharmacologist and psychotherapist to be in regular communication in order to differentiate between effects of medication and those of psychodynamic psychotherapy.

Annabelle's swings from anorexia to bulimia became greatly moderated after only several months in treatment and, in fact, were not seen by either of us as her major problem but rather as a part of her thought and behavior patterns constituting her anxiety, depression, and obsessional withdrawal from the world.

While the physician monitored Annabelle's vital signs, mood changes, and variations in anxiety, as well as persistence or relief of obsessive-compulsive behavior, as her psychotherapist I continuously evaluated her progress in terms of her ability to form a therapeutic attachment and do insightful work in therapy. As we have seen, many of those suffering from obsessive-compulsive disorders have difficulty forming therapeutic alliances or attachments, since their defense mechanisms are partially predicated on denial of the need for dependency and support. The more intense the level of anxiety, the more active the mechanism.

If the patient is distracted by obsessional thoughts, she is emotionally unavailable to the therapist, and he or she must be keenly sensitive to the patient's cues indicating such distraction within the session. In Annabelle's case, medication made her more accessible to therapy by reducing sufficiently her level of anxiety, panic, and depression for her to focus on her own dynamics and personal history. She could now distance herself from the activity of the disorder.

Sometimes the need for medication may be short-term, but nonetheless important. Psychiatric resident Lauren's symptomatic behavior (self-mutilation) disturbed her almost as much as the stressful states that led up to it. "It could drive me to do anything to myself to relieve it," she said. Some immediate relief was required. Lauren was referred to a psychopharmacologist who prescribed a tranquilizer and, with support from her friends, the immediate crisis subsided.

Often medication, although important when it is needed, may eventually be discontinued. This was true for Lara, whom we met in chapter 11. Following some two months of therapy, medication was prescribed, and it produced significant alleviation of her panic attacks. Although she still experienced panic, she was able to stay in control of her behavior. After two years the medication was tapered and discontinued, and no increase in agitation was noted.

Sometimes the best answer is no medication at all, despite appearances that might indicate the contrary. April was fifteen when she came to me. She had been discharged from a girl's boarding school as a result of her anorexia nervosa, low weight, and strange, nonsocial OCD rituals. Concern over her health by the school was the major reason for sending her home. She was thin, though not skeletal. Her five-foot-six frame weighed in at ninety-two pounds.

She was occasionally tense and even tearful when the subject of her relationship with her father came up. "He's just not there! He only talks about superficial things, and I see how he hardly talks to my mother. It's been like that for years! I know that my mother's upset about it and I hate to see her miserable. I wish she'd divorce him."

Apart from this painful issue, April showed no intensity, sadness, or anger about other concerns. When she described her eating rituals and her exercises (she ran five miles a day and did calisthenics afterward), she did not seem upset. Oddly enough, April seemed to be, in general, rather relaxed, yet she was compelled to follow a rigid pattern of behaviors and rituals each day.

Within only three months of outpatient treatment three times a week and no medication, April gained twenty-three pounds, reaching her goal weight of 115 pounds, and several months later gave up her rigid exercise routine in exchange for a more flexible one. She varied her eating pattern in addition to increasing her calories. She had several family-therapy sessions with one parent present at each. Confronting her mother about her "desperate marital situation," her mother indicated that it was far from perfect but also far from desperate. In a later session, April confronted her father about his superficial conversations, and he indicated his willingness to discuss any subject that she wanted to talk about. During these sessions, April was expressive and articulate about her feelings, crying and becoming angry at appropriate moments.

April had entered therapy eighteen months after the onset of observable signs of OCD and anorexia nervosa. She had seen one individual therapist and one family therapist before I saw her. I explained to April that people developed both OCD and anorexia nervosa as an attempt to stay balanced, to stay calm while being unable to depend on anyone else. I explained that she could now begin to use trust and dependency to stay on balance instead of the ideas and rituals she was currently using;

that I would help her gain weight without getting fat, and help her relinquish her rigid exercising without feeling chaotic.

April's progress was extraordinary, even for someone who had utilized these symptoms for only eighteen months. She made friends at a local school, developed a weekend social life, and was generally symptom-free and relaxed. Her ability to use supportive therapy to make progress swiftly ruled out the need for medication. The most significant clue to this was her calm, relaxed demeanor and the absence of complaints about mood and anxiety level.

Her illness was clearly a reaction to her family system and her inability to confront her parents with her unhappiness. This created a reactive anxiety that she controlled with OCD and eating-disorder defenses. Since she had no chemical disorder at work, April gave up her symptoms when the situation was cleared up by counseling and therapy.

The medication dilemma is complicated by the display of similar symptoms by persons suffering from different constitutional problems: depression, anxiety disorder, panic disorder, and mania. The severity and degree vary. Sometimes they are combined, making it difficult to determine if medication is necessary and, if it is, what the medication should be. Determining the nature of the interplay between constitutional, familial, and sociocultural factors requires a high degree of skill and experience on the part of the mental health practitioners involved. If medication is required, the psychotherapist must be on guard for symptoms of guilt or depression due to prolonged use of drugs.

Annie, a recent college graduate who was suffering from a severe depression that prevented her from functioning at her first job or from taking care of personal needs at home, began a course of antidepressant medication that improved her mood and stabilized her. After two months on medication, she came into therapy with a smile on her face. But when I asked how her week had been, her smile disappeared abruptly.

"I don't know why this happens to me," she said, becoming tearful, but continuing to talk while she cried. "I'm feeling good one minute and upset the next. This happens to me several times every day. I never know what mood I'm going to be in next."

"Does that mean the medication is no longer helping you?"

"Well, no, I . . . I stopped taking it nearly a week ago."

"And now—do you feel like you did before you began taking medication?"

"Yes, pretty much."

"Then you felt better when you were taking medication?"

"I guess that's right . . . but I just think that maybe it's not me when I'm on medication. I would just like to feel better without anything that alters who I am."

"But how are you managing without it?"

"I'm crying a lot and I feel like I'm losing control of myself, especially after work. There I stay pretty much in check."

"Then you feel more stable at work?"

"No! Absolutely not! I just keep myself under control until five o'clock, then I come home and either cry or eat until I nearly explode—or both. Yesterday I couldn't make it and luckily there was nobody in the ladies' room. I just kept washing my face with cold water until I could stop crying."

"Then you're not provoked into being upset by anything at work . . . or at home."

"Nope. It's just something within me. I guess it was always there."

"Does taking medication upset you?"

"Yes," she admitted.

"Why?"

She looked away as she answered. "When you first suggested it, and you wanted me to go for a medication consultation, I thought that you were trying to get rid of me, that you just wanted me on some pills so you wouldn't have to work so hard with me. That feeling went away. I can see that you're the same with me, but now I guess that I just resent taking pills just to be a normal person. Each time I take one, I feel reminded that something is wrong with me."

"You feel better when you don't take the pills?"

She smiled, then laughed. "When I don't take the pills, I *know* that there's something wrong with me."

"What are you going to do about this dilemma?"

"Take the pills and bitch about being defective, I suppose."

Annie's resentment of medication is typical. Her feelings of inferiority or defectiveness because of the need for medication certainly reflect our society's negative view of drug dependency. It took some time in therapy to reframe these attitudes and allow Annie to accept her need for biochemical assistance, just as a diabetic must accept her need for insulin, though unlike a diabetic, she may outgrow her need for medication.

Some patients are well aware of their dependence and attachment to their rituals, they clearly express a fear of losing them through medication because the rituals are a major part of their sense of self. This was the case with Paul, who exhibited severe cleanliness disorders, and who is discussed in chapter 6. After four months of treatment (with substantial progress), I requested that he try medication intended to reduce his obsessive-compulsive behavior, and he filled the prescription. When he came to my office for his next visit, I asked, "How is the medication affecting you?"

He looked embarrassed, then smiled and laughed nervously before he said, "Well, to tell you the truth, I haven't taken it yet."

"Oh? But I thought that when you saw the doctor for medication, you were anxious to begin."

He nodded. "I was. I'm really surprised at my own response. I did fill the prescription, but I looked at that bottle of medicine, and I thought about what would happen if I lost all my rituals, and even though I came here to get rid of them, when faced with the medicine that—maybe—would get rid of them at least partially, I was actually afraid to take it . . . I guess I just don't feel like I'm ready to get rid of them. I feel like I'll have nothing without them."

By the time Paul had been in treatment for six months (two months after the medication had been prescribed), he agreed to go on a very low dose of the medication to see what sort of effect it would have on him, and how he would deal with a diminished need to go through his obsessive-compulsive rituals. He did this and felt that his need diminished somewhat. He did not, at first, reduce his rituals; he just enjoyed knowing that he had a choice. He did not feel he could emotionally abandon them, but he liked the idea (it took some getting used to) that someday he might give them up.

Paul stayed on his half dose of medication and within six months managed to give up almost 75 percent of his rituals. The dose he was taking was far below the clinically recommended strength, so there is a real issue as to whether Paul was simply giving up the rituals and using the medication as a placebo, or whether he was very sensitive to it and was able to lose most of his symptoms with only a modest dose.

Now four years into treatment, without increasing his medication level at all (even taking it erratically), almost all of his rituals have disappeared, and he is doing very well. Paul prefers to believe that he, himself, has given up the rituals, and the medication was not responsible.

SIXTEEN

Hospitalization

If psychotherapy is sought too late, office visits, no matter how frequent and no matter how competent the therapist, may not be enough to deliver an individual from the dangers of obsessional conduct. The patient's life may become so organized around obsessive behavior that without it he or she will mentally disintegrate. In such cases, the need is for twenty-four-hour-a-day care offered by hospitalization.

The most frequent category of obsessional disorder that requires hospitalization is the eating-disordered patient. Severely emaciated anorexics, as well as chronic and endangered bulimics, are hospitalized due to the life-threatening nature of their obsessional symptoms. Before the public became aware of anorexia nervosa, often dubbed "the obsession that kills" in magazine articles, obsessionality, as characterized by obsessive-compulsive disorders, was considered little more than a relentless nuisance (handwashing being the most common example). It is the eating disorders that have focused attention on the severity of the problem and the need to successfully treat obsessional disorders.

Generally the patient with an eating disorder who enters a

psychiatric hospital has other problems as well. Typically, major depression and/or borderline personality disorders accompanying the eating disorder are seen. Some patients show both anxiety and panic disorders as well. In many cases, the eating disorder that prompted the hospitalization is secondary to one of the other disorders. With these patients, we see an even greater tenaciousness in their obsessionality to compensate for an even greater sense of emptiness.

A psychiatric hospital that treats anorexia nervosa or bulimia becomes aware all too quickly of the stubbornness of the patient's symptomatic behavior. Most hospitals utilize many staff members to thwart what can be life-threatening behavior. Inpatient care and management with the eating-disordered patient is very much like managing a chronically suicidal patient who has to be supervised continually to prevent self-harming behavior. But the program needs to be constructed so that restrictions on both the patient's behavior and the amount of privacy allowed can be removed as the patient relinquishes symptomatic behavior. Otherwise, the program becomes nothing more than well-organized coercion.

Hospitalized patients still need to negotiate the same conflicts that other obsessional patients in outpatient psychotherapy do. Thus the task of the psychiatric hospital is two-fold: to reduce self-harming behavior, and to engage the patient in treatment with a primary therapist and adjunctive therapists. While some patients will no doubt require medication to relieve anxiety or depression, the major task of the hospital is to keep the patient engaged in treatment. If the patient is coerced outside of the treatment alliance, she can simply exercise her ability to emotionally withdraw (a highly developed skill), and submit to the treatment only until she is discharged. At that time, symptoms generally reappear.

Psychiatric hospitals treat mental illness at its most acute stage, and in most cases only in its most acute stage. This poses special demands for the staff. They must learn to become fully invested in a patient even though the treatment may be of short duration and, perhaps at the most successful point in the therapist-patient relationship, she may be discharged. The staff should see their therapeutic goal as allowing the patient to learn how to trust, the understanding being that the hospital is preparing the individual for outpatient therapy and is a workshop in forming trusting relationships.

An example is the treatment given Debbie, whom we met briefly in chapter 4. When she came to the hospital, she had traveled a great distance because she believed (having phoned in advance) that the program would be helpful to her. So when she arrived for a screen interview, the admissions staff and I were surprised. Instead of meeting someone eager for treatment, we met someone withdrawn and reluctant. Debbie came into the office, took a chair near the window, looked out at the view, then pressed her forehead against the glass and said in a low voice, "Why did I come here?" This was her way of disenfranchising us as helping people.

"Since you called us," I said, "you probably had a reason. What was it?"

There was no answer, and we soon discovered that Debbie, like many OCDs, could both respond with and tolerate silence for much longer periods of time than was practical in the interview situation. The third of four children, twenty-year-old Debbie's infant care had been the responsibility of a young nanny who was constantly with her until the child was six years old. At that point, the twenty-four-year-old nanny abruptly gave the family two hours' notice and left with no forwarding address.

"Debbie just seemed to stop," her mother told me later. "She would walk around, looking confused and dazed all the time. She talked in school, but not at home."

Eventually Debbie became anorexic and bulimic. Now she was underweight, but not severely so, and not enough for it to be a health hazard. She was five feet six and weighed ninety-one pounds.

Once we got by Debbie's total silence in our first session, she explained to me that she always became intensely involved in whatever task she undertook. "I go to the limit," she said, "and even when I'm not doing the things, I can always think about them." In this way, she warded off feelings of emptiness and a failing sense of identity. She explained that she had coped this way since beginning elementary school. "I was always happier at school than at home. In school, I knew what I was supposed to do. School made me feel more adequate than home."

On her good days in the hospital, Debbie could be seen being cheery and playful with other patients and the staff as well. She was exceptionally intelligent and could mobilize herself to charm, entertain, and delight the unit. But this pleasant demeanor could suddenly dissipate if someone gave her a compliment about how well she was doing, as I did in our second meeting.

"Sure, sure," she said. "I guess that's what everybody wants from me." Her smile quickly turned to a frown of displeasure. "They just want me to shut up and not complain, and to keep smiling. Nobody ever wants to really know how I feel, which is that I'm a fake. I'm supposed to keep everybody happy. Well . . ." And now she was shouting. ". . . I hate it!"

Sitting in a straightback chair, she suddenly grasped the arms of the chair tightly, leaned her head forward and suddenly thrust it backward, slamming her head into the wall behind her. As she leaned forward to smash her head a second time, I jerked the chair forward, away from the wall. She thrust her head back quickly in an attempt to hit the wall before it was out of range, but it was now too far behind her. She looked dazed, then annoyed at having her behavior thwarted. She stood up, edging backward toward the wall. I grabbed her wrists and pulled her away from the wall before she could fling back her head again.

"Leave me alone!"

"No. I won't leave you alone! And if you don't stop this, I'll send for nursing and this session will be over."

She started crying. I was lucky, maybe today she would tell me why she wanted to bang her head.

"What are you feeling?" I demanded.

"You don't understand!" she shouted.

"Then tell me."

All the while, she looked forty-five degrees to either side of me or at the floor. "You don't understand. All I feel is empty! I don't feel like I'm anybody. I'm nothing!"

"Sit down." I motioned to the chair.

She did and resumed crying.

"Why were you banging your head?" I asked her.

"Because I could feel it! When I feel empty, I can't feel anything. I have to feel something."

Debbie was an overachiever. When her obsessional defenses worked, she was able to achieve her goals in school-related tasks, but when stress overwhelmed the pseudo-identity derived from her achievement-oriented behavior, she experienced a dissociative state. She termed it not being able to feel anything. She then organized around the pain generated from her head banging. This brought her back from a feeling of mental annihilation.

Debbie was in frail balance. She demonstrated rigidity about routines, her personal care, her meals; even her walk was a measured gait. She was perfectionistic. She set unrealistically high goals for herself academically and then withdrew from courses when she thought she might not get an A. She made precise and perfectionist demands about her weight and her shape. She continuously belittled her appearance, declaring, "My thighs are too fat. No matter how skinny I get, my thighs never get thin." She would talk negatively about her facial features, her hair, nearly every aspect of her appearance. And the negativity extended to her personality as well. When discussing herself, she would remark, "I know that I'm selfish and greedy. I want too much attention. I would probably never be satisfied."

Because she viewed herself as totally negative, Debbie shied away from compliments or expressions of support from staff or patients, and was most comfortable when she adopted the guiding or supportive role herself. In this way she presented herself as a reluctant patient pursued by the staff, thereby provoking the rejection and abandonment that she felt had been her lot in life. The hospital staff understood that Debbie, underneath her rejecting behavior, secretly wished for connection and attachment to others. Staff members took turns talking to her for months, alternately confronting her about her acting-out behavior, inviting her to depend on them, and to join the rest of the patient community, which was genuinely interested in her. Debbie, in turn, alternately isolated herself and joined in and laughed with the rest of the patients in the unit.

While the staff behaved in a nurturing and structuring way, Debbie, when she had the courage to, behaved spontaneously, played at sports, games, and discussion, then alternately withdrew to obsessive-compulsive behaviors and head banging. Gradually, due to the staff's relentless efforts, Debbie engaged less in withdrawal and more in socially connected behaviors. She formed attachments to several patients and four staff members, the first time she had ever done so (according to records of her previous four hospitalizations and her family history).

The psychiatric hospital for Debbie had to form a sociofamilial milieu, so that she could develop dependency and accept limits from those she was reliant upon. The ability of a psychiatric hospital to form and maintain effective milieu therapy depends upon the size, training, and commitment of its staff to the concept of a therapeutic energy system. Since patients are both needy and demanding, there are few therapeutic shortcuts possible.

SEVENTEEN

Recovery

Earlier, I mentioned the pediatrician who was so moved when he first saw Nina. Standing in the doorway of her room, he watched her for some ten minutes, folding and refolding her clothing over and over, and he was stunned and shaken that she did this sort of thing all day long.

This pediatrician would probably be an apt spokesman for any parent who has watched a child go through the rituals involved in obsessive-compulsive disorders. It is simply heartbreaking to watch someone desperately repeat the unnecessary to the point where little else can be done with their daily lives.

Watching these individuals—whether children or adolescents or young adults—family members are not only deeply saddened, they are also antagonized, angered, and frustrated. In many cases, family members fear their own impulse to shout at the person, "Stop! This is crazy!" or shake them. They worry that any attempt to interfere might only make matters worse. So they often settle for retreating from the sufferers, despairingly watching them go through their useless behaviors again and again.

Do you remember the family of Emily? They were very

different from Paul's family. In her case we saw a family constructively interfering, and this involvement produced great progress. In Paul's case, we saw family members in effect enabling the OCD behavior to grow and take over his life. There can be no doubt what this implies for those who are living with and caring for victims of OCD, or what it implies for the sufferers themselves. But how is one to begin this process of constructive interference?

In chapter 1, I presented an anatomy of OCD. Let me now offer the same for treatment.

ANATOMY OF TREATMENT FOR OCD

1. Inviting dependency.
2. Unmasking rituals.
3. Talking in depth.
4. Regulating anxiety.

Before briefly reviewing these four areas, it should be made clear that I am not suggesting that OCD sufferers and their families take a blueprint from here and set out alone in search of recovery. The guidance of a well-trained therapist is essential. And even if it were not, the care and nurturance necessary to recover someone from OCD is more than that available within a family. For that reason alone, one needs to recruit either an individual therapist or a family therapist, or ideally both. Only with this guidance and support should the journey toward recovery be started.

INVITING DEPENDENCY

The individual who has descended into the ritualistic world of OCD has given up on others emotionally. Attempting to create the accessibility needed to invite dependency is no easy task. What will a person find attractive enough to make interference acceptable?

One of the things sufferers will find alluring is confidence. They must see in the family member or the therapist the kind of confidence that assures them of continuing (long-term) support and comfort. All sufferers of OCD are secretly wishing for someone who can intrude in their system, someone so attractive to them that they would be willing to negotiate and mediate their system in exchange for a sound relationship. In effect, they seek the kind of confident, authoritative person whose absence originally caused the sufferer to turn to rituals.

The role that sufferers themselves have in this area of their recovery process is the willingness to take a risk emotionally: the risk of trusting, of depending, the kind of gamble probably given up long ago. If they are suffering from OCD, it very likely has been a long, long time since anyone's voice calmed them down, since anyone's advice relieved them, since anyone's guidance made them hopeful.

In fact, they discarded others long ago in terms of their usefulness to them; and while discarding them, they said many things to themselves, such as, "No one else can understand. No one else can help me. No one else realizes how important all these ideas are to me. I have to do everything for myself. I'm the only one who can do them correctly. I'm the only one who can do things in a way that satisfies me."

Of course, the catch is that OCD sufferers *never* satisfy themselves, they never do it well enough, and, in fact, their thought processes are an endless repetition exactly like the rituals they perform.

So now their first task in attempting recovery is to understand that they have become so emotionally separate that others have been useless to them. They must once again make people valuable and important to them. They must let themselves *depend* on others.

UNMASKING RITUALS

A major part of engaging OCD sufferers in the treatment process will be getting them to talk about their rituals, but not too quickly, not as one might recite a menu or a shopping list. This must be far more than simply a recitation. Sufferers must be able to offer their secrets in a trusting relationship, and they must know that the helper realizes this is important information and must be treated accordingly.

This process can be difficult for many OCD sufferers. Discussing the rituals, after all, takes some of their magic away. It also makes the sufferer vulnerable to arguments about the secret rituals, even vulnerable to ridicule in moments when members of the family become frustrated. But these are all risks that must be taken to create real relationships, to create something interpersonal, to create something that is not the kind of separateness that is termed obsessional.

Talking in Depth

Unless care is taken, discussing the rituals, much like doing them, can become only a way to avoid facing something much more basic: the underlying hopelessness and despair of dependency, the sense of chronic anxiety, never-ending mind racing, and separateness that first gave rise to the rituals.

If you are a family member, getting a sufferer to discuss these deeper issues will be extremely difficult. If you are a therapist, it will be a bit easier, for you will not feel the pain to the degree it is felt by a family member trying to treat a relative. The therapist does not have to contend with the heartbreak that such a discussion engenders, and the sufferer does not have to contend with as much embarrassment when speaking to a therapist.

REGULATING ANXIETY

Once the treatment process has begun in earnest, both thera-pist and family should seek alternative ways for the sufferer to cope with anxiety. An examination of job and marital status, lifestyle, where a person lives, all aspects of a life need to be explored in terms of improving the environmental aspects of that person's life. What part of the day-to-day conditions creates anxiety for this person? Is there a way to change jobs? To live in a different location? These could be very helpful in reducing the anxiety that drives OCD.

In the instance of a young child or an adolescent suffering from OCD, what we want to look for are outside forces that detract from the family's cohesiveness and its ability to provide adequate nurturing. We even need to look at community cultural issues, which sometimes conspire to separate members of a family from each other.

A second area to explore concerning anxiety is relationships. Is there something helpful that might be done with parent-child or spousal relationships or even friendships? If we are dealing with a young adolescent, do we want to change that person's school to one where the sufferer could relate better? Have others in the environment detected that the sufferer is unusual, thus closing off that environment socially? All rela-tionships should be explored to see how they can be improved.

And the third area that has to be considered is what can be done, if anything, with pharmacological intervention. Some individuals will need none at all, some will need a period of many years of medication, some may need a lifetime. It is impossible to suggest one kind of care for all sufferers. Cer-tainly, medication to regulate anxiety is something that should be considered.

* * *

This, then, is the Anatomy of Treatment—the process of exchanging ritualistic behavior (which is nondependent and therefore obsessional) for depending upon others (which, while it may be needy, is not obsessional). But it must be stated here that treatment should not be approached with unrealistic hopes for a quick recovery. On the contrary, expectations should be for a long-term process.

Of course, if an individual has shown obsessive-compulsive behavior for only six months or a year, that is a wonderful sign, for it is not seriously chronic and perhaps with short-term treatment and family work the symptoms will disappear. But this is not the most likely situation. Since OCD is often kept secret for months and even years, when family members first notice it—when they first *know* they are seeing it and are determined to do something about it—the rituals are already well entrenched, and they have a tenacious quality. If, for example, someone has practiced rituals for a number of years, they have become part of the person. They are not so much seen as a disability or illness, they are simply seen as one facet of a person's personality, and they will likely take several years to begin to diminish.

Any mention of a time table for recovery is purely speculative, but it is a healthier and better strategy to expect it to take a longer rather than a shorter time. If an attempt at treatment is made with high hopes for a quick recovery, and it does not happen, there will be a new despair settling over the sufferers and their families, and this can only reinforce the despair that may have sparked this illness in the very beginning.

So the process will be long and difficult. But what matters most is that recovery *can* be achieved. Those of us who have been fortunate enough to see the dramatic success that is possible—to watch a Paul begin to feel again or an Olivia begin to trust and depend again or a Nina begin to eat and speak and live again—know that the potential reward is well worth the effort.

That pediatrician who was moved to tears when he first

observed Nina in her room also saw her just before she left the hospital. "You can't put a price tag on that," he told me. "She was just doing the kinds of perfectly normal things any kid does, but it was the most beautiful sight in the world."

INDEX

Abandonment, fear of
  in children of alcoholics, 142
  and hospitalization, 126–27, 175–176
  as major impediment to psycho-
    therapy, 81–82, 83, 91, 96
  resulting from parentification of
    child, 118
  and therapist's reassurances, 98,
    102, 109, 133
  see also Dependency
Addiction, food. *See* Bulimia nervosa
Addiction pattern, 66
Aggression, 56, 57
Agoraphobia, 73, 162
Alcohol, abuse by bulimics, 65
Alcholics, children of, 47–53
  as adults, 52–53, 141–42
  anxiety of, 49, 51
  breakdowns of, 51–52
  compensatory behavior by, 47
  defenses of, 48
  distrust of, 51
  nuturance drain on, 47–48, 51, 52,
    53

self-destructive behavior by, 49,
  50, 52, 53, 141–142
therapeutic treatment of, 49–53,
  141, 142
therapeutic treatment obstacles, 51
therapeutic treatment turning
  points, 53, 141
Ambivalence, 33
Anger, 136
Anorexia nervosa, 55–64
  atypical, 43, 148
  causes vs. consequences, 57
  compared with bulimia, 65–66
  control issue, 56–57
  and defensive denial, 109
  and developmental emptiness, 32–
    33, 36–37
  and eating rituals, 145, 148, 149,
    150
  family frustration with, 59
  and fashion-model ideals, 22, 26–
    27
  hospitalization for, 171–76